Anthony Fusimate

W. T. HOLLINGER

W. T. HOLLINGER

A GUIDE TO PATHOLOGICAL EVIDENCE

by

FREDERICK A. JAFFE

M.D., M.Sc.

Director, Department of Laboratory Medicine,
Queensway General Hospital, Toronto.

Former Medical Director, Centre of Forensic Sciences,
Province of Ontario.

Consultant Pathologist, Toronto Western Hospital,
Consultant Pathologist, Forensic Associates,
Assistant Professor, University of Toronto.

THE CARSWELL COMPANY LIMITED

Toronto, Canada

1976

©The Carswell Company Limited 1976
ISBN 0 459 31640 0

TO THE MEMORY OF
DORIS AND ALEXANDER

PREFACE

Q. "In your career I have no doubt you have from time to time been
   engaged on one side or the other of litigation with some other
   distinguished doctor on the other side?"
A. "Yes."
Q. "And the side that you have been engaged on has been represented
   by counsel—I am sure by eminent counsel—and during his cross-
   examination of the expert on the other side, have you sometimes
   wished you were doing it yourself?"
A. "I have sometimes wished I might have conducted it."
Q. "And in fact, there cannot be any very profitable examination of
   an expert except by an expert?"
A. "I think that probably in the majority of cases that can be said . . ."

This passage taken from the cross-examination of pathologist Dr.
James Webster by Mr. Maurice Healy K.C. during the trial of
Frederick Nodder* conveys the purpose of this book. In a subject like
forensic medicine to which many excellent textbooks, originating from
both sides of the Atlantic, are devoted, a writer must justify the
addition of yet another volume.

Both in giving evidence for the prosecution and in advising the
defence I have often found that the difficulties experienced by
counsel and the court lay not so much in the unfamiliarity of medical
language or even in the complexities of pathological concepts as in
an insufficient understanding of the scope, and therefore the limits, of
the pathological investigation itself. The pathologist, on his part, like
other expert witnesses, is inclined to assume that his special knowledge
is so beyond the comprehension of lay persons that his findings and
opinions will be accepted without serious challenge.

The biological material with which the pathologist has to deal will
often, even under the most favourable conditions, not permit conclusions which leave no room for doubt. By pointing out, therefore,
the uncertainties which are inherent in even the most competent
examination, this book hopes to put the role of the pathologist into
perspective, to make his evidence more meaningful to the non-expert
and to expose it to greater scrutiny.

No attempt has been made to cover forensic medicine in breadth

---

*Duke, Winnifred (ed.), *The Trials of Frederick Nodder, the Mona Tinsley Case*,
Notable British Trials Series, Vol. 72, p. 161. London: William Hodge & Co., 1950.

or in depth and the matters discussed are merely those which most often arise in court. The writer's experience at the City Morgue of Metropolitan Toronto and at the Centre of Forensic Sciences of the Province of Ontario forms the basis of the book, but many others have contributed to it.

I am greatly indebted to Mr. D. M. Lucas, Director of the Centre of Forensic Sciences, for making available to me the incomparable resources of this institution and for permission to include Figs. 2-1, 7-1, 12-4 and 13-2. Mr. George Cimbura, Section of Toxicology, Mr. R. C. Nichol, Section of Firearms, and Mr. Elgin Brown, Section of Biology, were kind enough to review parts of the manuscript and to give me the benefit of their expert knowledge.

It is also a pleasure to thank Miss Lana Thompson for her technical assistance and Miss Laura Ball, Librarian, for her invaluable help in obtaining many of the references. Mr. U. von Bremen and his associates of the Photography Service of the Centre generously contributed of their time and skill.

My colleagues, Dr. Marvin Smout of London, Ontario, and the late Dr. John Penistan of Stratford, Ontario, reviewed the entire manuscript. Their constructive criticism resolved many ambiguities and enhanced the usefulness of the book.

I am most grateful to Mrs. Kristina Blum of The Carswell Company for bringing about the difficult metamorphosis of the manuscript into the book.

Mrs. Dorothy Irwin drew Fig. 8-2 and my son Charles Fig. 1-8. My secretary, Mrs. Barbara Gardner, typed parts of the manuscript.

Without my wife's constant encouragement the book would never have been completed. Many of her suggestions were incorporated into the text and her talent for detecting flaws in grammar and syntax found much application in the reading of the notes.

It lies in the nature of medico-legal work that autopsies often have to be performed at inconvenient times and under difficult conditions. I would be remiss if I did not acknowledge with gratitude the skillful assistance I received over many years from morgue attendants Mr. George Duncan and the late Mr. Christian Heck.

F. A. J.

CONTENTS

1

THE MEDICO-LEGAL
AUTOPSY

Religion and magic are the remote ancestors of both medicine and law. Their slow and uneven evolution into separate realms of knowledge has become a fascinating part of man's cultural history. In spite of their gradual divergence, a common concern remained in such matters as violence and death, pregnancy and legitimacy, poisons and insanity. These areas of common interest, however, did not begin to emerge as a distinct subject until the end of the sixteenth century, and its final acceptance as a specialty, marked by the establishment of professional chairs at some European universities, had to await the beginning of the nineteenth century. Even today it is difficult to define its precise limits, or even its substance, and this is reflected in the multiplicity of the names by which it is known.

The term "Forensic Medicine" is generally applied to those parts of medicine which are employed in the solution of legal problems. Many medical specialties like pathology, psychiatry, obstetrics and serology thus have "forensic" applications. "Medical Jurisprudence", often used interchangeably, should designate those parts of the law which are concerned with the practice of medicine. "Legal Medicine" is used, particularly in North America and the Latin countries, to refer to the entire domain of common interest.

"Pathology", although meaning literally "the knowledge of disease", in its modern sense comprises that branch of medicine which studies the tissue changes caused by disease, ageing, violence or poisons. Its practice is not confined to the performance of autopsies but includes, in a clinical environment, the examination of tissue specimens taken from living patients for diagnostic purposes.

The autopsy, also called necropsy or post mortem, has as its main objective the determination of the cause of death. When performed for medico-legal purposes it may, in addition, have to establish the human origin of the remains, the identity of the deceased and the circumstances under which death occurred. It always comprises a naked eye (gross) examination but the condition and completeness of the remains determine what further steps will be taken.

When dealing with intact bodies the external inspection is followed by the removal and gross examination of the internal organs, usually supplemented by weighing and measuring. The microscopic study of tissue samples is nowadays considered an integral part of the post mortem examination.

Depending on the type of case, the autopsy may entail the recovery of bullets or other foreign objects, the procurement of tissues or body fluids for chemical analysis or serological testing, the taking of photographs or x-rays and the collection of hair samples, vaginal washings or fingernail scrapings.

The main concern of the legal authorities is the immediate cause of death and the detection or exclusion of the effects of violence. The interest of the pathologist, on the other hand, goes beyond this. He must, during the fleeting moment of the autopsy, identify those conditions which led to death, but he must also assess to what extent other, often unsuspected, injuries or pathological conditions may have contributed to the outcome and what the effects of medical treatment have, or might have been.

He is aware that any omissions on his part may not be remediable and that his conclusions, which may guide the police investigation, may have a decisive impact upon the liberty and reputation of others. He knows that every aspect of his conduct may be questioned in court and that his conclusions, and even his competence, may be tested by searching cross-examination. His task is made more difficult by destructive processes some of which were initiated by death itself (post mortem changes), others caused by external agents such as insects and animals. During all this time he may be under great pressure to produce early and definite answers to questions posed by the police investigators and he may have to explain to them that autopsies do not always yield results as unequivocal as might de desirable.

The signs and the diagnosis of death

Death is the irreversible loss of those properties which are the manifestations of life such as growth, movement, metabolism and reproduction. In a complex organism like man, death occurs in two stages. During the first stage (somatic death) the circulatory, respiratory and nervous systems cease to function and the body is no longer an integrated whole. It is this stage of somatic death which extinguishes the personality and constitutes legal death.

Cells, or even whole organs, may survive for several hours depending on their oxygen requirements, but eventually these too die (cellular or molecular death).

This distinction between somatic and cellular death was of mere philosophical interest until it became possible to maintain the circulation and respiration artificially and in this way to postpone somatic death and until the transplantation of organs demanded their removal from the donor prior to cellular death.

The traditional definition of somatic death, which was the complete and permanent cessation of circulation and respiration, therefore had to be modified to include the function of the brain. (See "Sydney-Declaration" in the Glossary.)

Many of the classical tests for the presence of death are more picturesque than practical. The cutting of a large artery, for instance, which is still recommended in many textbooks, to see whether the circulation has stopped, may be dramatic (especially if the person is not dead!) but is hardly advisable. The circulation may be assumed to have ceased if there is no pulse, heart beat, blood pressure or electrical activity in the heart (electrocardiogram) during a 15 minute period.

The absence of chest movements, breath sounds (as detected by placing a stethoscope over the larynx) and air movement through the mouth and nostrils indicates absent respiration.

The loss of nervous activity causes lack of reflexes, flaccidity of muscles and cessation of electrical brain activity (electroencephalogram).

The size of the pupils, which in the past has received much attention, is of no significance. Not only do the pupils dilate and subsequently contract after death, but they remain reactive to locally applied drugs, but not to light, for some time.

The diagnosis of death may be made erroneously in conditions which depress respiration and circulation. Notorious amongst these are overdosage by opiates and barbiturates, electrical shock, fainting (syncope), near-drowning and shock in infants after a difficult delivery. Such mistakes are especially likely if the examination is done in distracting surroundings, like heavy traffic.

The popular interest in such cases is largely due to the fear of premature burial. While in a modern environment premature burial is very unlikely, the erroneous diagnosis of death may well result in the omission of resuscitative measures which could have preserved life.

Post mortem changes

Following somatic death the body's defensive mechanisms break down and a number of physical and chemical processes (post mortem changes) commence which eventually lead to complete disintegration of tissue and cell structure. The body cools rapidly, reaching equilibrium with the surrounding temperature within 48 hours. The circulation ceases and all cells are subjected to lack of oxygen (anoxia). Those which are most dependent on oxygen, namely the cells of the brain, succumb first while less sensitive cells, like those of muscle and connective tissue and sperm cells, may survive for several hours.

The early breakdown of the tissues is due to the ferments (enzymes) normally present in them. Later bacteria, largely originating from the gut, the respiratory system and the vagina, also play an important part (putrefaction).

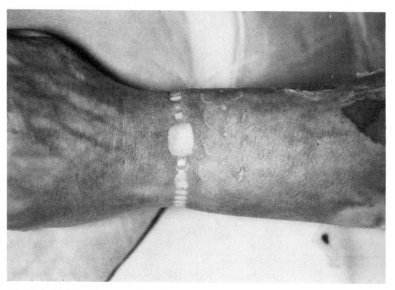

Fig. 1-1. Lividity does not develop in areas in which the blood vessels of the skin are compressed.

Post mortem changes are of great interest to the pathologist because they

    (1) confirm the fact of death,

    (2) provide a rough indication of the time of death,

    (3) may indicate that the body has been moved after death,

    (4) may reflect the cause of death,

    (5) may be mistaken for pre mortem lesions,

    (6) rapidly destroy signs of soft tissue injury and many features upon which the establishment of identity is based.

The most important post mortem changes are summarized in Tables 1-2 to 1-6.

Table 1-2
Post mortem cooling

Description

The gradual fall of the internal body temperature to that of the environment.

Mechanisms

Radiation is the main mechanism in exposed bodies. Evaporation is significant in damp or wet bodies in which it may temporarily lower the body temperature below that of the environment. Conduction is the chief manner of heat loss in submerged bodies and the only mechanism of heat loss from the interior of the body.

Progress

The body surface begins to cool immediately after death and feels distinctly cool after 4 hours. The fall of the internal body temperature, however, must await the establishment of a temperature gradient towards the surface and may thus remain unchanged for 1 to 3 hours. Complete temperature equilibrium is usually attained after 48 hours.

Modifying conditions

Clothing, bedding, a large body mass (obesity) retard cooling as does an external source of heat (sun, radiator). A small body mass (infants) and immersion in water favour cooling. Heat loss by radiation increases with the temperature difference between body and environment and also depends on the effective radiating surface of the body.

Forensic applications

The internal body temperature is the single most useful measurement upon which an estimate of the time of death may be based during the first 15 hours. If possible, several successive readings should be taken while the body remains undisturbed at the scene. Its usefulness is impaired by the fact that the body temperature at death is usually unknown and by the many modifying conditions.

Table 1-3
Hypostasis

Description

The pooling of blood in the vessels of the dependent parts of the body. In the skin these parts become dark red or reddish-blue (lividity).

Mechanism

The lividity of the skin appears within the first half hour after death and is at first entirely due to distension of capillary blood vessels by blood (hypostatic or congestion lividity), but after about 8 hours hemoglobin begins to diffuse into the tissues (diffusion lividity). At first the distribution of lividity may be altered by changing the position of the body but as diffusion lividity increases the lividity becomes progressively more "fixed".

Modifying conditions

Lividity will not appear in areas in which the capillaries are compressed as in weight bearing areas or in areas of constriction (Fig. 1-1). It is faint or absent in death preceded by large blood loss. Deep skin pigmentation tends to obscure it.

Forensic applications

The lividity of the skin reflects the colour of the blood and may thus indicate certain forms of poisoning (e.g. carbon monoxide). Hypostasis in internal organs may be mistaken for pathological conditions such as pneumonia. The location of lividity may occasionally indicate that the body has been moved after death. Patches of lividity must be distinguished from bruises, if necessary by microscopic examination.

Table 1-4
Rigor mortis

Definition

A transient stiffening and shortening of muscles which follows the state of primary flaccidity. Muscles in contact with a hard surface show flattening.

Onset and duration

Inconstant. Generally appears 2 to 3 hours after death, becomes generalized in 6 to 9 hours, remains generalized 24 to 48 hours, then gradually disappears.

Distribution

First observed in the face and jaw, then in the upper limbs, last in hips and legs. Disappears in the same sequence. This anatomical sequence has been attributed to differences in muscle mass.

Mechanism

Not known. The onset of rigor mortis and its development parallel certain chemical changes.[40, 97]* Its regression is accompanied by an increase in muscle ammonia.[154]

Variants

Muscle groups or the entire musculature may show rigor immediately after death (instantaneous rigor, "cadaveric spasm"). This tends to occur when death was preceded by violent exertion or emotion. Rigor has been reported at delivery of stillborn infants. Goose flesh is a manifestation of rigor of the hair muscles of the skin.

Modifying conditions

Violent exercise immediately prior to death and a high body temperature hasten the onset and spread of rigor. Stretching of a muscle abolishes rigor completely or partially depending on the degree of stretching and stage of development of rigor.

Rigor mortis must be distinguished from stiffening due to heat, which is permanent, stiffening due to freezing which disappears on warming, and the rigidity of the limbs due to the accumulation of putrefactive gases.

---

*References are to the Bibliography beginning at p. 159.

Table 1-5
Putrefaction

Description

A phase of rapid disintegration of the body accompanied by the production of gases. The skin and the hair and nails become detached. The internal organs gradually lose their integrity and become converted into a semi-liquid mass.

Mechanism

The chemical basis of putrefaction is the breakdown of proteins by bacteria. Most of these bacteria come from the intestine but others may enter through wounds. Ferments from insects and insect larvae may also play a part. Putrefactive gases are mainly hydrogen sulphide, ammonia, methane and carbon dioxide.

Progress

The appearance and rapidity of putrefaction depend greatly on the environment. The earliest changes are usually visible after 48 hours and gaseous distension is prominent after one week. Putrefaction gradually ceases after 6 to 8 weeks.

Modifying conditions

Conditions favourable to putrefaction include an abundance of bacteria, a suitable temperature, moisture and air. Both immersion in water and burial tend to retard putrefaction by lowering the temperature while in the case of burial exclusion of air is an additional factor. The bodies of newborn infants putrefy slowly because of lack of intestinal bacteria.

Effects of forensic importance

The gasses will distort the facial features making visual identification difficult. The swelling of the body may lead to an overestimate of body weight and will lower the specific gravity so that submerged bodies rise to the surface. The post mortem diagnosis of air embolism will no longer be possible and the flotation test of the lungs of newborns becomes invalid. Fermentation of sugars may result in the formation of ethyl alcohol.

Table 1-6
Adipocere

Description

A waxy, friable substance derived from the fatty tissues. It is usually greyish-white but may absorb pigments from clothing or the soil. Its odour has been described as "sweetish", "rancid" or "offensive".

Distribution

Under favourable conditions all fats in the body may undergo conversion into adipocere but the change is usually most marked in the subcutaneous tissues.

Chemical and physical characteristics

Adipocere is largely a mixture of crystals of free fatty acids. Owing to its low specific gravity it floats on water. It fluoresces under ultra violet light. It is insoluble in water but soluble in fat solvents.

Formation

Adipocere is the result of the hydrolysis of neutral fats by tissue and bacterial ferments. A moist environment is favourable but sufficient water may be derived from the tissues themselves.46

Time of appearance

This varies greatly with prevailing conditions, especially the temperature. In a cool environment 4 to 6 months are required for adipocere to become apparent but in a hot climate the time may be much shorter. Under favourable experimental conditions it may be seen microscopically after 7 days.

The role of the attendant

The role of the autopsy attendant, who is still occasionally known by the old German designation "diener", is not formally delineated and depends to a large extent on his experience and the confidence the pathologist has in him. He is responsible for guarding the body against unauthorized interference, for the maintenance of the morgue and the autopsy premises and for the care of the instruments. He will place the body on the table and, after the completion of the autopsy, close the body, return it to the storage facility and subsequently release it to the undertaker.

The attendant is generally permitted to make measurements and weigh the body and may be asked to be a witness to the formal identification procedure. He will usually keep a register of autopsies, of personal effects removed, of specimens taken and of their disposal.

While the services of an attendant are of great help to the pathologist, carelessness on his part could easily raise doubts about the validity of the pathological evidence. The testimony of pathologists has been successfully attacked when it was shown that attendants had undressed the body and removed the contents of pockets before the arrival of the pathologist, had washed the body, had used disinfectant or deodorant sprays or solutions in the room or had made incisions or removed organs in the absence of the pathologist.

Sources of error

The medico-legal autopsy is a complex operation, often lasting several hours, and frequently performed in unsuitable surroundings and under great pressure. Errors committed during its performance naturally detract from the value of the findings and the validity of the pathologist's opinion.

The autopsy is basically a destructive procedure during which the body cavities are opened, the relationship of organs irretrievably altered and appearances changed. Certain observations must be made at definite stages of the autopsy, otherwise such omissions cannot be remedied. If, for example, the interior of the chest cavities was not examined immediately after they had been opened and blood was subsequently allowed to escape into them, it would no longer be possible to say whether they had contained any blood originally.

Most of the common errors are avoidable and have as their common denominator the inexperience of the pathologist. They include:

(1) The performance of an incomplete examination (failure to examine the brain or to inspect the back).

(2) Inadequate documentation (omitting the recording of weights or measurements, or the taking of photographs or x-rays).

(3) Recording the findings too long after the autopsy.

(4) Removing skin deposits by washing the body.

(5) Failure to take appropriate samples for chemical analysis or taking samples improperly (unsuitable containers, inadequate labelling).

(6) Accidents during the autopsy (dropping specimens on the floor).

(7) Mistaking iatrogenic, post mortem or autopsy artefacts for significant lesions.

(8) Reluctance to enlist the help of experts in other forensic sciences.

(9) Placing too much reliance upon preliminary information concerning the identity or cause of death.

The destruction of the body by decomposition and external agents will rarely mislead the experienced pathologist but will, by obliterating evidence of disease and signs of soft tissue injury, severely limit the information the autopsy may yield.

Table 1-7

Common surface injuries

	Description	Causation
Abrasion	an injury to the surface of the skin	
graze		a rough surface
imprint		localized pressure
scratch		a pointed object
Avulsion	a tearing away of a part or tissue	a heavy object (*e.g.*, a tire) passing over the body
Blister	a collection of fluid underneath the superficial layer of the skin	heat, skin diseases, infections, drugs, poisons, putrefaction

	Description	*Causation*
Bruise	a hemorrhage into the subcutaneous tissues	blunt force, blood diseases
Contusion	an injury to a tissue without disruption of the surface	blunt force
Cut	an incised wound, longer than deep	a sharp object
Laceration	a crushing or tearing of tissue, showing a break in the surface	many types of violence
Split	a longitudinal laceration of the skin	compression of the skin between bone and a hard object or surface
Stab	a penetrating wound, deeper than wide.	a pointed object

Terminology

Some terms, while not peculiar to forensic medicine, are either used more frequently than in other fields or have acquired special meanings. Some of these are illustrated in the following diagram. Only those which are likely to give rise to misunderstandings will be briefly discussed.

Survival time

This is the time interval between receipt of the lethal injury and death and it may range from a fraction of a second to several years. Questions concerning survival times frequently arise in court because of the following:

(1) If the time of death is known, an estimate of the survival time may indicate when the lethal injury was sustained.

(2) A survival time of several hours may permit the partial or complete elimination of drugs or poisons.

(3) A long survival time may permit partial or complete healing of injuries.

(4) A very long survival time, e.g. several years, may raise doubts concerning the role of the supposedly lethal injury in the causation of death.

(5) In a case showing several potentially lethal injuries an estimate of the survival time of each may indicate the sequence in which they were sustained.

(6) The performance of voluntary acts by the victim requires a certain minimum survival time.

(7) In situations in which several individuals sustained lethal injuries simultaneously, an estimate of survival times may suggest the sequence of deaths.

As the above shows, an accurate knowledge of the survival time would often be crucial, but this the pathologist can rarely have. He must instead rely upon the tissue changes of vital reactions and healing, upon certain chemical findings, upon his knowledge of the fate of ingested drugs and poisons but mainly upon his general experience with trauma. The great individual variation in the reaction to injury will always put the pathologist who estimates the survival time on uncertain ground.

Post mortem interval

In many criminal and civil proceedings the time of death becomes of importance and an estimate of the post mortem interval, that is the time span between death and the examination of the body, has to be made. The difficulties inherent in this are discussed in the section on "Time of Death" in Chapter 2.

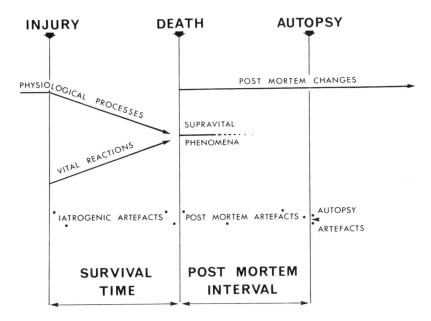

Supravital processes

These are physiological and pathological processes which continue beyond the point of somatic death, mostly at the cellular level. Their forensic usefulness is limited.

The best known are the supravital processes in the gastro-intestinal tract. It is generally agreed that after death food does not leave the stomach nor move along the intestine. Supravital digestion of food, on the other hand, may progress to a signifcant degree, eventually destroying the wall of the stomach or intestine itself. It is this supravital digestion which makes the state of the food in the stomach such an unreliable indicator of the time of death, even if the time and nature of the last meal are known.

Engulfment of small inhaled particles by certain cells in the lung may occur for several hours after death and is commonly seen in cases of drowning or smoke inhalation.

The growth of hair and fingernails, however, which has been said to occur after death belongs to the realm of folk lore.

Iatrogenic artefacts

These may be pre mortem in origin such as operative incisions, needle marks, defibrillator marks and broken ribs inflicted during heart massage, or post mortem such as the absence of organs removed for transplantation. A new iatrogenic condition is now appearing in patients who had been maintained on a respirator for long periods and who show marked swelling and softening of the brain. Some of the common iatrogenic lesions which must be distinguished from the effects of violence are shown in Fig. 1-8.

Post mortem artefacts. Autopsy artefacts

In addition to the usual post mortem changes, bodies are subject to many destructive influences. Those floating in water or exposed to heat are particularly likely to show post mortem alterations. During transport abrasions or impressions of ropes or straps may be inflicted or stomach contents may be spilled into the mouth or upper air passages. In soft tissue lacerations a paucity of bleeding and the absence of a cellular reaction, as shown microscopically, are indicative of a post mortem origin. Recently the activity of tissue ferments has been studied. Post mortem wounds showed a complete absence of ferment activity, although even vital wounds required a period of several hours before ferment activity became demonstrable.[48, 145]

Likely to cause more difficulty is the destruction caused by animals and insects. These are especially likely to attack external wounds such as lacerations, cuts or bullet wounds and quickly make their nature unrecognisable.

Artefacts caused by the embalming process and by the autopsy itself pose special problems. The most important autopsy artefacts, which have on occasion misled the pathologist, are hemorrhages in the muscles of the neck and air bubbles in the veins of the surface of the brain. The former may become very important in cases of suspected strangulation. It is, therefore, essential that during the patho-

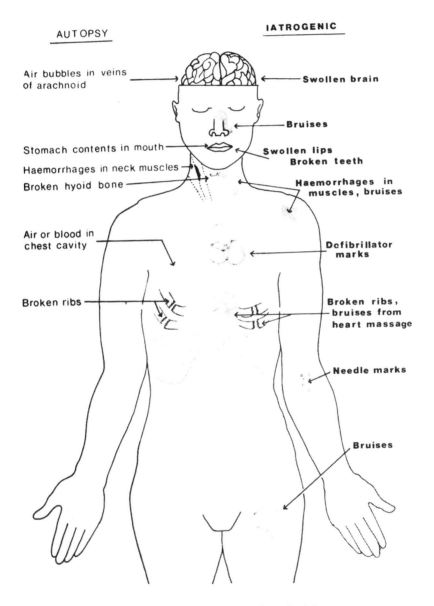

Fig. 1-8. Common findings of artefactual origin.

logical examination certain precautions be taken to prevent their occurrence because once such hemorrhages have been caused, they are indistinguishable from pre mortem hemorrhages.

Photography

The great value of photography in the documentation of a case lies in the fact that, as the autopsy progresses, appearances are inevitably and irretrievably destroyed or distorted. Blisters break, lividity fades and veins distended with air collapse when incised. Certain injuries, moreover, such as bite marks on the skin, can only be accurately recorded by means of photographs while still in situ.

The number of photographs to be taken varies from case to case and largely reflects the interest of the examiner. In cases of assault, photographs should be taken before and after undressing the body, as well as before and after any washing.

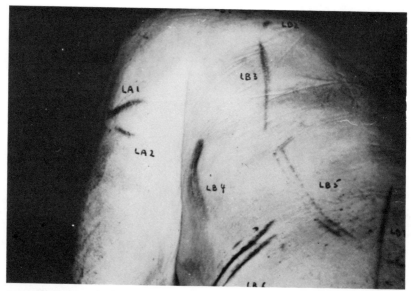

Fig. 1-9. Annotated photograph of contusions of the trunk and arm inflicted by beating with a rifle barrel.

Colour photography is excellent for general documentation and for teaching purposes, but courts have been reluctant to admit colour photographs in evidence fearing their emotional impact on the jury. Certainly, almost all findings could be adequately shown in good black and white prints except, of course, such matters as the subtle differences in colour between bruises of various ages, which would make colour photography essential.

Photographic prints which accompany the autopsy protocol and which illustrate several lesions should be annotated. A suitable code e.g. LA for left arm, LB for left side of back etc. can easily be devised. In referring to the lesions the text of the protocol should, of course, employ the same code. A typical annotated photograph is shown in Fig. 1-9.

A scale should be shown in all close-up photographs. In investigations involving several bodies a name or number tag identifying the particular body should appear in every picture.

Authority to perform autopsy. The pathologist's responsibility

The authority to perform a medico-legal autopsy is derived from a judicial source such as a coroner, crown or district attorney or medical examiner. In many jurisdictions this takes the form of a warrant which not only confers the necessary authority but places the pathologist under a legal obligation to carry out the duties involved.

Having received such authority, the pathologist is in sole charge of the medical investigation. He will decide its scope and hence must bear the responsibility for any inadequacies or omissions. In addition to the actual dissection his duties include the description of the findings, the taking of photographs, the securing of specimens for expert study, their proper packaging and their submission to the laboratory in such a manner that the continuity of the evidence is not destroyed.

Also implied in the authority is both the right to retain the body until all medical studies have been completed and the obligation to guard the body against any wilful or injudicious tampering.

As fresh bruises may not become visible on the skin surface for some time after death (Fig. 4-3) it is good practice to retain the body in cases of assault or "hit and run" accidents in order to give the pathologist the opportunity for a "second look". The increasingly common practice of retaining a pathologist to advise defence counsel makes it proper, at least in major criminal cases, to keep the organ or organs upon which the diagnosis of the cause of death had been based. This would give the opposing pathologist an opportunity for an independent examination.

Attendance at the autopsy

While it is not advisable for the pathologist to be alone during a medico-legal autopsy, the attendance should, for practical as well as esthetic reasons, be restricted to those who perform a relevant function. These may include, apart from the pathologist and his assistants, the coroner, investigating police officers, photographers, forensic scientists and, on occasion, the undertaker or cemetery officials. Anyone acting on behalf of the defence should, of course, be admitted but his function should be strictly limited to that of an observer. Relatives, the public and newspaper reporters must be excluded.

A list of those who were present during the autopsy should form part of the protocol.

"Identification"

Before the autopsy can commence, a formal "identification" of the body must be made. This may be done by a relative or friend of the deceased directly to the pathologist in the presence of witnesses or indirectly through a police officer or morgue official. Naturally, the fewer persons involved the better. In any event, the "identification" should be made by someone who would be available for any subsequent trial or inquest.

The term "identification" is unfortunate because it implies the establishment of the identity of the deceased. Actually, the identity will often be unknown; in fact, the purpose of the autopsy may be to establish it. The formal "identification" therefore, may not be made by name but merely by designating the body as that found at a certain time and place. The purpose of the formal "identification" is to preserve the continuity of evidence and to establish in court that it was upon a certain body, and no other, that the post mortem examination was performed.

Clothing

The expert examination of the clothing does not fall within the bounds of the medical examination, but the pathologist is responsible for its removal from the body and its submission to the laboratory. It may become of great importance in cases of doubtful identity as well as in cases of assault, rape, shooting and stabbing.

All items of clothing and jewellery should be briefly described and any disarray recorded, preferably photographically. The description should indicate whether buttons were done, undone or missing, zippers closed or open, shoe laces tied and belts buckled.

The clothing should be removed from the body without cutting or tearing. If cutting is unavoidable, care must be taken not to cut through any tears, stains, bullet holes etc. Clothing must never be allowed to fall on the floor.

Each article of clothing or jewellery should be put into a separate plastic bag and labelled. Unless it can be taken to the laboratory very quickly, moist clothing should be air dried before packaging. No attempt must be made to clean it by brushing or washing as this may remove important trace evidence.

Visiting the scene

The activity of the pathologist at the scene of a death is largely limited to the taking of body and environmental temperatures. Nevertheless, the impression he may gain of the body and its surroundings, the state of the clothing, the distribution of blood stains etc., will be much more meaningful to him than any information he may receive second hand. It follows that the pathologist who encounters the body for the first time in the morgue, as often happens, starts his examination at a disadvantage.

The performance of the forensic autopsy

External examination. Very little may be known about the deceased or about the circumstances under which death occurred, so that the external examination is much more important in a forensic case than in a hospital autopsy. Even trivial injuries may become very significant (Fig. 9-2).

After the body has been weighed and measured, a general inspection is carried out followed by a detailed examination of each body region, starting at head and progressing downwards, including the back. The presence and distribution of lividity and of rigor mortis are noted. The body's state of nutrition and cleanliness are described and whether its appearance corresponds to the given age.

The body temperature may be taken but this is rarely of value once the body has been transported to the morgue and is, of course, quite meaningless after refrigeration.

Odours, while often unpleasant to the bystander, may be of great help to the investigator. Alcohol, phenol, paraldehyde, cyanide and Oil of Wintergreen may be detected in this way and this is one of the reasons why disinfectant or deodorant sprays must not be used in the room.

Old amputations, malformations, birth marks, scars and tattoos are recorded. The latter, being usually voluntary and decorative, convey much about the personality and interests of their bearer. Involuntary tattoos are much less common and are mostly seen in drug addicts in the form of small dark dots caused by the use of sooty needles.

Stains, vomitus or crystalline deposits on the skin are collected either by swabbing or scraping. If signs of decomposition are present these are described in detail and samples of insect eggs, maggots or pupa cases are retained for further study in the laboratory.

Fingerprinting, the collection of fingernail scrapings, hair samples and vaginal washings, the taking of anal swabs and the excision of bullet wounds and needle tracts are also best done before the body is opened.

The importance of an adequate description of all external injuries, even those seemingly trivial, is self evident. Annotated photographs (Fig. 1-9) are invaluable. The possible appearance of bruises some time after death must be remembered.

Accurate measurements of surface injuries are important, especially as imprints may indicate the dimensions of the injuring object. In the recording of bite marks great precision is essential and this can be accomplished only while they are still in situ and the body surface undisturbed.

When an injury of the scalp is found, the surrounding hair must be shaved in order to obtain a clear view of it. Any description of a scalp laceration in which this was not done must be regarded with suspicion.

The precise location of each injury should be determined by measuring its distance from the nearest heel or from another anatomical landmark such as the nipple or the umbilicus.

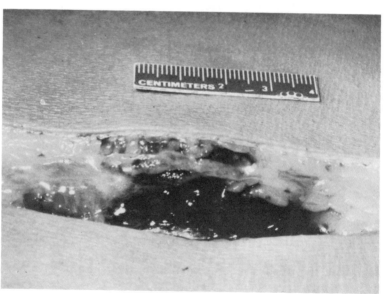

Fig. 1-10. Even large bruises of recent origin may not be visible on the skin surface.

If it is decided to x-ray the body, this should also be done before the internal examination is commenced. Fractures of the limbs, the nose, the neck and the skull are often apparent externally but their precise nature and extent can best be shown radiologically and by exposing them during the later stages of the autopsy.

Internal examination. The sequence of the steps involved in the internal examination depends to a large extent on the personal preference of the pathologist and on the type of case. They always include the opening of the skull and the body cavities and the inspection of the organs in situ followed by their systematic removal and detailed naked eye examination.

The dissection is usually commenced by the making of a Y-shaped incision on the front of the body, extending from the tip of the shoulders to a mid-point over the centre of the breast bone and from there to the public region. This type of incision may have to be modified in order to prevent it from passing through wounds.

In fresh bodies this initial incision usually yields sufficient blood for alcohol analysis. This method of obtaining the blood sample prior to the opening of the body cavities forestalls any subsequent allegation that it may have been affected by diffusion of alcohol from the stomach and reduces the chance of contamination by yeast organisms.

If the chest (pleural) cavities are to be examined for the presence

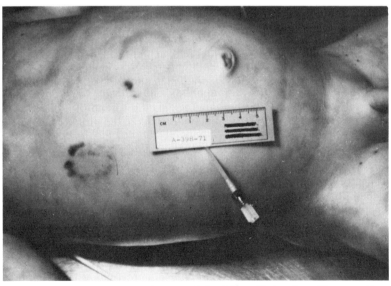

Fig. 1-11. Bite marks must be recorded while still in situ. (Courtesy Dr. I. Ramzy.)

of air (pneumothorax), this must be done at this stage by puncturing the chest wall under water. Once the pleural cavities have been opened the presence or absence of air can no longer be ascertained.

The contents of the chest and abdominal cavities are then examined. Stab wounds and bullet tracts must be explored before the relationship of organs has been disturbed and blood vessels must be inspected for air embolism before they are cut.

The removal of the heart usually yields a large amount of blood which is suitable for toxicological analysis and blood grouping but which should not be used for alcohol determination.

The entrance (esophagus) and outlet (duodenum) of the stomach are tied before its removal to prevent loss of stomach contents. In cases of suspected poisoning the intestine may be tied at intervals and the contents from its various portions collected separately.

During the removal of the organs samples of tissue, such as liver, or of body fluids, such as bile or urine, may be taken for analysis and blocks of tissue for microscopic examination. Whether a microscopic examination is actually carried out again depends on the type of case and the interest of the pathologist. It is the only way to recognise or to exclude many disease processes and is still the best method of estimating the age of injuries.

The examination of the head begins with the reflection of the scalp. Bruises, which may be visible only on its deep surface, may indicate the number and direction of impacts. In removing the skull cap the use of hammer and chisel should be avoided as these may produce fractures. The dimensions and contours of depressed fractures of the skull must be recorded with precision as they may be the same as those of the object which caused them.

The examination of the neck is usually postponed until the chest cavity and the skull have been opened. This relieves the congestion of the blood vessels of the neck and reduces the chance of producing artefactual hemorrhages which would not be distinguishable from those produced by pre mortem violence.

It is usually not necessary to remove the spinal cord except in cases showing injuries to the spine and in cases of "battered" children.

The autopsy protocol

This is the final written record of the pathological findings and forms the permanent basis on which the medical aspects of the case may be judged. Unlike the evidence given verbally in court which must be kept brief and in terms understandable by laymen, the autopsy protocol is a scientific record. Medical terminology is used and accuracy is not sacrificed for brevity. Negative findings, while omitted as much as possible from oral evidence, are fully recorded in the protocol.

The text of the protocol should consist almost entirely of a purely factual description of the findings. Opinions and interpretations should be confined to the final summary. It is in this final summary that any unusual features of the case or any unresolved questions are discussed.

The exact format of the protocol is largely determined by the preference of the pathologist but the following list includes its usual sections:

(1) Name and age of deceased

(2) Description of body at the scene

(3) Time and place of the autopsy

(4) Authority by whose order the autopsy is being performed

(5) Persons attending

(6) "Identification" of the body
    (a) Time, date, place
    (b) Name of person making the "identification" and his relation to the deceased
    (c) Names of witnesses

(7) Description of clothing

(8) External appearance of the body

(9) Gross internal findings

(10) List of specimens retained
    (a) Type of container, seal numbers
    (b) Date, time and place of their disposal and names of persons receiving them

(11) Photographs
    (a) List of photographs
    (b) Name of photographer

Later may be added the following:

(12) Microscopic examination

(13) Results of laboratory examinations

(14) List of diagnoses
    (a) Principal diagnosis first, others in decreasing order of importance

(15) Summary
    (a) Opinions concerning the cause of death and the circumstances under which it occurred
    (b) Uncertainties, discrepancies
    (c) Persons consulted and their opinions

(16) Signature of the pathologist

Table 1-12

Matter which fall within the scope of the pathological examination	*Matters usually referred to experts in other forensic sciences*
Examination of skeletal remains	
Description of injuries. Human origin, number of individuals, body stature, age of juvenile remains, "lying age".	Bone fragments, sex characteristics, age of adult remains (anatomist, radiologist). Racial characteristics (physical anthropologist).
Dental examination	
General description and charting of dentition. Retention of dentition and dentures. Recording of bite marks.	Detailed study of dentition and dental work, study of individual teeth, sex and age characteristics of teeth, comparison of bite marks with dentition of suspects, interpretation of dental x-rays (forensic odontologist).
Sexual assults	
Description of clothing and injuries, collection of vaginal washings, clothing, hair samples. Microscopic examination for sperm cells.	Blood and seminal stains, blood groups, acid phosphatase, hairs, fibers (biologist). Hair for trace elements (physicist). Sexual personality disorders (psychiatrist).
"Hit and run" accidents	
Description of wounds including tire marks, collection of glass, paint, chromium fragments.	Paint, glass, chromium fragments (chemist, motor vehicle expert). Identification of tires (motor vehicle expert).
Deaths due to firearms	
Number and direction of shots, recovery of bullets, bullet fragments, wads etc. Matching of holes in clothing with wounds. X-rays of body. Excision of entrance wounds. Microscopic examination of tissues.[135]	Characteristics of weapons and ammunition, test firing of suspect weapons, examination of deposits around entrance wounds (ballistics expert). Trace metal deposits on skin or clothing (physicist). [96, 133]
Poisoning	
Clinical course and tissue changes of poisoning. Collection of pocket contents, samples of tissues and body fluids for analysis.	Collection of pills, powders etc. at the scene (police). Chemical properties of poisons, analytic methods and their sensitivity and specificity (toxicologist).

2

QUESTIONS
THE PATHOLOGIST
TRIES TO ANSWER

The condition of the body as disclosed by the post mortem examination represents the final outcome of those injuries or diseases which caused death. In addition, it demonstrates the stage which the individual's growth and aging processes have reached, often other injuries or pathological disorders not directly related to death and the effects of medical treatment. The recognition and distinction of all of these may be made more difficult by a large variety of artefacts and post mortem changes. From his findings the pathologist must deduce the events which preceded and finally led to the terminal state, a task which has been compared to the reconstruction of a film sequence from the last frame.

Some common questions which arise at autopsies are discussed below. It will be seen that the answers the pathologist can give must often be less complete or precise than might be desirable. Deaths which occurred under certain special circumstances pose peculiar problems and require specific methods of investigation. These will be reviewed in subsequent chapters.

Are the remains human?

When whole organs, teeth, hair, finger or toenails, portions of skull or intact long bones of adult individuals are present the recognition of their human origin is no problem, but when dealing with fragmentary remains or those of infants or young children difficulty may be encountered.

Serological tests, which are highly specific, may establish the origin of fresh tissue or blood. These tests, however, depend on the preservation of tissue protein which putrefaction and high temperatures quickly destroy. Freezing and drying at room or outdoor temperatures, on the other hand, may preserve these proteins and may make serological testing possible even after months or years.

Especially demanding may be the examination of remains recovered after a fire. Not only is the degree of destruction often very great and serological testing not possible, but the remains of animals are frequently intermixed with those of human origin.

How many individuals do these remains represent?

This question most often arises following disasters, such as aeroplane accidents or fires, when exhuming remains from mass burial sites and when examining dismembered bodies.

When dealing with skeletal remains only a duplication of specimens, such as several left thighbones is an absolute indication that more than one individual is represented, but marked differences in the size of bones, age or secondary sex characteristics naturally suggest a multiple origin.

When soft tissue is also available the organs may indicate individuals of different sex or different blood groups.

When the pathologist is provided with only small specimens of soft tissue, especially if decomposing, or if only small bone fragments are recovered, the number of individuals represented often cannot be determined.

Whose body is this?

The establishment of the deceased's identity is part of every medicolegal autopsy. There may be little difficulty with fresh bodies on which a relative or friend may make a direct visual identification. Identifications on the basis of scanty remains, on the other hand, belong to the most formidable problems in forensic medicine.

The establishment of identity takes place in two phases which in practice often overlap. The first, which might be called the "general" identification establishes the type of individual with regard to sex, body build, age and race. It is based solely upon the autopsy findings. The second phase, the "specific" identification, aims to establish the person's individuality and involves a comparison of the autopsy findings with records of an individual made during life. It thus depends on the existence of such records, be they photographs, dental charts, fingerprints or x-rays. In their absence no specific identification may be possible.

Items used in general identification:

Sex	Eyes
Age	Teeth (general)
Race	Hair
Body length	Parity
Body weight	Blood group

Items used in specific identification:

Facial features	Scars, signs of surgical
Fingerprints	operations
Teeth (details)	Fine bone structure
Birth marks	Skeletal abnormalities
Tattoos	Lip prints

As the disintegration of the body progresses many of these items become obscured and the identification more difficult until, in the case of skeletons, only the dental data and bone findings are available.

There can, of course, never be absolute certainty in any identification because there is no theoretical reason why two individuals could not have the same physical characteristics, dental work or even fingerprints. In practice, however, the probability of this occurring, especially when there are many points of comparison, becomes so small as to be negligible.

Of great value in both phases of the identification are the clothing, the personal effects found in pockets or near the body, and jewellery, but the possibility of planned deception must always be kept in mind. When the feet are intact, measurement from the heel across the sole to the tip of the second toe will indicate the shoe size while, conversely, the size of the shoe will indicate the size of the foot which, in turn, will suggest body stature.

Much of the information which may lead to the establishment of the identity, such as stature, weight, sex and age may be gained during the usual autopsy. Cases of exceptional difficulty may require special methods of investigation, some of which fall outside the realm of pathology and belong to such fields as forensic odontology or physical anthropology, but the pathologist who is cognizant of these methods will not fail to secure those specimens on which they depend.

Facial features. Unfortunately, the facial features which are both the most distinctive and the most easily recognized personal characteristic, are rapidly distorted by post mortem changes and destroyed by animal or insect action. In well preserved bodies frontal and profile photographs should be taken as soon as possible. The thickness of the soft tissues over the various parts of the skull has been studied and, based on such data, plasticine reconstructions of the face may be attempted. This method, however, is difficult and, in the present state, belongs to the art, rather than the science of medicine.

Fingerprints. The taking of fingerprints, which is usually done by the police, remains possible as long as the outer layer of the skin (epidermis) is present. In fresh bodies this is no problem. In decomposing bodies or in those in which drying of the fingertips has occurred, the fingertips may have to be amputated and submitted to the laboratory for restoration and printing. Even in extensively burned bodies there may be sufficient preservation of skin to make fingerprinting possible (Fig. 7-1).

Lip prints. These have not yet been used widely, except in Japan, but appear to be as individual as fingerprints.[183]

Tattoos. These are located in the deeper layers of the skin (dermis) and remain distinct even in the presence of moderately advanced putrefaction. Closeup photographs should be taken or the tattoos removed and preserved in formalin.

Sex. The external genital organs of both sexes are rapidly affected by putrefaction and insect infestation. The prostate gland, however, and the non-pregnant uterus resist decomposition for a long time. Even when these can no longer be recognised grossly they can often be demonstrated microscopically.

As long as the cell nuclei can be stained, attempts can be made to determine the sex of the tissues by finding certain structures in these nuclei. The so-called "sex chromatin" or "Barr body" represents one of the X chromosomes and is indicative of female cells. This finding has even been made in the cells of hair roots in the examination of single hairs.[123]* More recently the "fluorescent body" or "F body" which represents the Y chromosome and is indicative of male cells has been used. This method seems applicable to blood stains[21] as well as to cartilage and bone marrow.[15]

Skeletal characteristics. X-rays of the skeleton, apart from showing major abnormalities like fractures, may reveal the details of fine bone structure, such as the location of blood vessels and the internal (trabecular) architecture of bone. These may be very important in the second phase of the identification, provided that comparable x-rays taken before death are available for comparison.

Teeth. The study of the teeth (forensic odontology) is an essential part of every autopsy on an unidentified body. While its main value lies in the establishment of the identity of the deceased by comparing the post mortem dental findings with dental records made during life, even a preliminary inspection may give indications of age and, with a lesser degree of certainty, of the sex, social group and geographic origin. While the general pathologist should hesitate to embark on forensic odontology, he should, nevertheless, be able to record the dental findings in such a manner that they could, if necessary, be evaluated by an expert in forensic odontology.

Comparing bite marks with the dentition of suspects will rarely fall within the responsibilities of the pathologist. For a fascinating example of such evidence the reader is referred to the account of the Biggar murder.[77]

---

*References are to Bibliography beginning on page 159.

The pathologist should secure all loose teeth and retain all dentures and denture fragments. The teeth should be inspected and the location of cavities, location and type of fillings, caps, bridgework etc. recorded on a dental chart. Dental x-rays serve not only as a permanent record of the dental findings but, especially in the younger age groups, are the best means of assessing tooth development. If the body is likely to remain unidentified for some time, the entire dentition should be retained (Fig. 2-1).

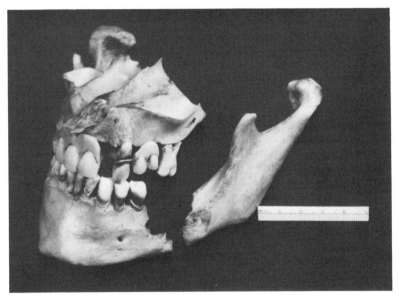

Fig. 2-1. Retained dentition including a partial denture. The defect in the lower jaw represents a bullet wound.

The role of the expert in forensic odontology, who usually has a professional background of dentistry or dental surgery rather than of pathology, includes, apart from the study of bite marks, the assessment of age, sex, racial characteristics and the recognition of dental methods and materials peculiar to certain parts of the world.

For an excellent account of the scope and methods of forensic odontology see Gustafson.[71]

The time of death

No problem in forensic medicine has been investigated as thoroughly as that of determining the time of death on the basis of post mortem findings. Apart from its obvious legal importance, its solution has been so elusive as to provide a constant intellectual challenge to workers in many scientific fields. In spite of the great effort and ingenuity expended, the results have been meagre.

In theory, it should be possible to use either vital processes, such as the growth of the beard, which are terminated by death, or those changes which are initiated by death. The latter have received the most attention. Ideally, the phenomenon, whether physical or chemical, should be measurable so that it could be mathematically related to time. It is clear, however, that time is only one factor which governs the progress of post mortem changes and that the conditions under which the body had been lying, its physical characteristics and the circumstances under which death occurred are at least as important. The relative effect of these other factors becomes greater as time elapses and thus the determination of the time of death becomes progressively more imprecise.

Body temperature. This is still the most useful single indicator of the time of death during the first 15 hours. After this period every degree of temperature decline corresponds to ever increasing time intervals and the method becomes increasingly inaccurate.

It is the internal body temperature which must be measured and this can be done by the insertion of a thermometer into the rectum or the abdominal cavity. The accuracy of the method can be improved by taking successive temperature readings at known time intervals, but during this entire procedure the body should not be moved nor its attitude changed, conditions which could only rarely be fulfilled in practice.

The loss of heat from the body, especially from its interior, is a more complicated process than had been believed. As heat loss occurs only on the body surface and as heat from the interior can reach the surface only by conduction, the internal body temperature does not fall significantly for some time after death. This "temperature plateau" generally lasts ½ to 1 hour but may persist as long as 3 hours.[158] For a discussion of the physical principles involved in the cooling of the body see Marshall.[110, 111, 112]

The following table giving examples of cooling rates is taken from Marshall:[112]

Cooling rates (°F per hour) for the extended unclothed adult body in an environment of 60°F

Body Build	Thin or Small	Average	Fat
During first 3 hours	1⅓	1	5/6
next 3 hours	2⅔	2	1⅔
next 3 hours	2⅓	2	1⅔
next 3 hours	1⅔	1½	1⅓
Between 12-15 hours p.m.	1⅓	1½	1⅓

Note that the cooling curves illustrated in the above table are not exponential in nature (resembling the letter L) but, due to the initial temperature plateau, sigmoid (resembling an inverted S) in shape. Marshall recommends that the rates be reduced by one third in the case of clothed bodies and that a further reduction of up to 25 per cent be made for more compact attitudes of the body such as crouching. For a further discussion of post mortem cooling see Table 1-2.

Rigor mortis. This cannot be regarded as a reliable guide to the time of death except within very wide limits. In the case of a body lying undisturbed at room temperature, if rigor has not yet appeared the post mortem interval is probably less than three hours, if rigor is generalized 10 to 48 hours and if it has completely disappeared probably more than 60 hours. In exposed bodies, particularly if subjected to low temperatures, the limits are even wider. See also Table 1-4.

Lividity. This appears within the first 30 minutes. It becomes progressively "fixed" during subsequent hours due to intravascular coagulation of blood and diffusion of hemoglobin. See also Table 1-3. It is too variable to serve as an indicator of the time of death.

Changes in the gastro-intestinal tract. The estimation of the time of death based upon the degree of digestion of stomach contents is a time-honoured one, but one which involves so many uncertainties that it has been largely abandoned. Even when the time and nature of the last meal are known, the physical and emotional state of the individual prior to death, the type of physical activity, the thoroughness of chewing etc., all influence the rapidity of digestion. In addition, significant post mortem digestion may occur.

The stomach emptying times are very much subject to the same sources of error as the assessment of the degree of digestion, except that food does not leave the stomach after death. Generally, a meal has left the stomach after 4 hours but emotional disturbances may cause considerable delay. While the type of food eaten is no doubt important, the great uncertainty in the field is reflected in the discrepancies between published stomach emptying times. For instance, the emptying times given for eggs range from 2 hours, 40 minutes to 3 hours, 30 minutes, for vegetables from 2 hours, 15 minutes to 3 hours, 30 minutes and for veal from 3 hours, 30 minutes to 5 hours, 30 minutes.[79, 175]

Passage through the intestine. The head of a meal passes through the small intestine at a rate of 6 to 7 feet per hour hour, reaching the large intestine in about 3 to 3½ hours. As the contents of the small intestine are semi-liquid in consistency it may not be possible to recognize the head of a meal unless it is of a distinctive colour or contains undigested elements such as grains of corn. Again, many intangibles, particularly emotional factors, may affect the passage of intestinal contents.

Changes in the eyegrounds. Kevorkian[92] studied the changes in the eyegrounds during the immediate post mortem period. During the first five minutes there is segmentation of the blood column in the blood vessels of the retina and other changes occur during the next 7 to 10 hours. The quantitative evaluation of these changes requires considerable experience and it is likely that their main value lies in the recognition of clinical death rather than in the estimation of the post mortem interval.

Insect infestation. Exposed cadavers are likely to be infested by many types of insects ranging from the two-winged flies (diptera) which lay their eggs on the body a few hours after death, to a variety of mites and beetles which participate in the terminal disintegration of the body after putrefaction.

The study of the entomology of the cadaver received its impetus through the work of Mégnin[118] at the end of the last century, but the hope that it might provide a reliable guide to the time of death has not been fulfilled. Most of the studies have been devoted to the flies because these are prominent in the early post mortem period and because the growth of their larvae can easily be observed in the laboratory. The occurrence of certain flies in a given locality, the time in which their eggs hatch and the growth of larvae, however, are dependent on so many geographic and climatic factors that even an expert entomologist can provide only a very rough guide.[102]

The many other methods which have been used in attempts to determine the time of death include the irritability of muscle,[142] the reaction of the pupils to drugs[9] and the movement of sperm cells.[101] None of these have achieved even the modest success of the methods discussed above.

The cause of death

The belief is common amongst the public that the pathologist, having performed a post mortem examination, must have found the cause of death, a belief which is constantly being reinforced by novels and the entertainment media. Certainly, whenever a severe recent injury is found to have involved a vital organ, the causal relationship is not difficult to see. The pathologist is on almost as sure a ground when, examining a skeleton, he finds a severe pre mortem bone injury, such as a depressed fracture of the skull, and from this concludes that there must have been injury to the underlying organs.

In many instances the sequence of events is not as direct or as certain. Multiple injuries may have been sustained, none of them lethal in itself, but having a cumulative effect. The consequences of injury may have been aggravated by pre-existing disease or an injury may have initiated a long sequence of complications which finally led to death. An example of the latter would be a burn of the body surface which became infected and led to blood poisoning (septicemia). This in turn caused the deposition of infected blood clots on the valves of the heart (bacterial endocarditis) one of which broke off, was carried in the blood stream and blocked the main artery to the small intestine (mesenteric embolism). Following this blockage the intestine became gangrenous and this caused fatal inflammation of the abdominal cavity (peritonitis). Such a chain of events always raises the question concerning the role of the initial injury, especially as a very similar course could be initiated by non-traumatic disease.

Generally, the longer the survival time and the more complex the clinical course or the medical treatment, the more difficult it is to define the precise role of the initial trauma.

As will be shown in subsequent chapters, the detectable signs of lethal injury may be very inconspicuous or entirely absent, so that the diagnosis may have to be inferred from suggestive findings or from circumstantial information. Finally it should be emphasized that the discovery of a potential cause of death may not be the same as having found the cause of death.

Where did death occur? Has the body been moved?

The place of death is often unknown when bodies are recovered from rivers or lakes or washed ashore but rarely can the pathologist be of much help. The hope that in drownings the examination of the water in the lungs might provide a clue has not generally been realized in practice. The investigation of the surroundings of bodies found on land is largely a matter for the police but the pathologist should collect any material such as dust, leaves or grease which adheres to the clothing or the skin and should obtain fingernail scrapings.

Rigor mortis, which is the stiffening of the musculature and the flattening of muscles which have been in contact with a hard surface, is marked and generalized for 24 to 48 hours during the early post mortem period. If the body is moved during that time and placed in a different position, this is easily detectable because muscles which had been in contact with a hard surface remain flattened. Once rigor mortis has passed and secondary flaccidity has supervened this evidence disappears.

Lividity of the skin surface is absent in areas on which the body weight had been pressing. Once the lividity has become "fixed", a change in the position of the body can readily be detected (Fig. 8-1) but eventually putrefaction will obscure lividity.

Who died first?

In multiple fatalities, determining the sequence of deaths may be essential for the reconstruction of an accident or assault and may have important implications in civil law, but this is often easier said than done. The assumption that two bodies which had lain in the same environment would have undergone changes at the same rate and that, therefore, differences in their condition at the time of examination would reflect differences in the time of death, can be accepted only with many qualifications. Even small modifications of the local environment, e.g. a nearby radiator, could greatly influence the cooling rate and thus the progress of post mortem changes.

A simple example may illustrate the difficulty of the problem. Two persons who died in the same room of carbon monoxide poisoning were found to have blood carbon monoxide concentrations of 65 per cent and 75 per cent. At first sight, it may seem that the former must have died first, but as Graph 5-4 shows, by a more strenuous activity the second individual could have attained the higher concentration sooner. An uneven distribution of carbon monoixde in the room and, largely conjectural, differences in individual susceptibility to lack of oxygen add further uncertainty.

The nature and severity of any injuries and the performance of voluntary acts by the victims will have to be taken into consideration in assessing survival times and thus the probable sequence of deaths. In any event, the more closely the deaths followed one another, the more difficult and uncertain the determination of their order.

How old were the injuries? Which came first?

The pathologist is often asked how long before death a certain wound was sustained but his opinion can rarely be more than a rough estimate.

Only when it was of such severity that it must have caused death quickly does the injury itself indicate its time of infliction. When living tissue is injured certain changes take place in the area of injury, provided there is sufficient time, and it is upon this "vital reaction" that the pathologist must base his estimate.

The following example illustrates the reaction to a contusion of moderate severity. The disruption of tissue structure and the breaking of blood vessels occur at the time of impact and bleeding occurs into the tissue spaces. The amount of bleeding, its rapidity and its effect on the victim naturally depend on the number and type of blood vessels broken. The area will swell and become discoloured, although the swelling may not reach its maximum for 10 to 12 hours and the discolouration may not become visible on the skin surface for a day or two.

In very mild trauma only fluid, without red blood cells, may escape into the tissues leading to swelling without discolouration.

A certain type of white blood cell (polymorphonuclear leucocyte, fortunately generally known as "poly" or "polymorph") appears in about 8 hours and quickly becomes more numerous. As this type of cell normally occurs in the blood stream and therefore in the original hemorrhage, it is not its mere presence but its abundance which is significant. These "polys" begin to disintegrate in about 18 hours and this is followed by the breakdown of the red blood cells which begins after about two days and is complete in 10 days.

The red pigment (hemoglobin) is liberated into the tissues as the red blood cells break down and is transformed into small, brown, iron-containing crystals (hemosiderin). These can be demonstrated microscopically after about 5 days.

A second type of cell (macrophage) appears on the scene during the third day and begins to clean up the site of injury by engulfing cell débris and hemosiderin crystals. Fine yellow crystals of bile, which do not contain iron, can usually be found after 10 days.

These microscopic changes are reflected in the naked eye appearance of the area which changes from reddish-blue to blue to brown to green to yellow, fading gradually.

If the injury caused tissue disruption, the earliest signs of healing, in the form of proliferating fibrous tissue cells, are usually noticeable after three days and over the next few weeks this progresses to scar formation.

While these events permit a rough estimate of the time elapsed, other factors may modify this sequence and introduce further uncertainty. These include a break in the skin surface which would expose the wound to infection and to drying, the age of the individual and poorly understood differences in biological responsiveness. Relative dating, that is deciding the sequence of injuries in a given individual, avoids the last two variables and is, therefore, on somewhat firmer ground than absolute dating.

Putrefaction rapidly obscures both the gross and the microscopic signs of vital reactions and eventually precludes both absolute and relative dating.

The imprecision which is inherent in these methods has led to attempts to use the activity of various tissue ferments (enzymes).[145] It seems that some changes may occur as early as one hour after injury. These methods, however, are technically demanding and are, so far, largely based on experimental animal data. To what extent these methods will be applicable to practical forensic problems is still uncertain.

Were the injuries sustained before or after death?

It is widely believed that injuries sustained after death do not bleed while those sustained pre mortem do, but this is an over-simplification which could lead to serious error. Blood vessels are tubes which may contain fluid blood for some time after death. When blood vessels are broken, blood escapes into the tissues provided there is a slight pressure gradient from the vessel to the tissue, a condition which is fulfilled in areas of post mortem hypostasis or lividity.

As the pressure gradient after death is usually not great, hemorr-hage is usually not extensive and tissue swelling does not occur. In areas in which even small hemorrhages may be of great significance, as in the muscles of the neck, the distinction between pre and post mortem hemorrhage may not be possible.

A hemorrhage or bruise located outside an area of hypostasis must therefore antedate death, unless it can be shown that the area had at one time been the site of hypostasis.

The finding of hemosiderin, a white blood cell reaction or healing, of course, clearly mark an injury as pre mortem.

Enzyme methods[48] promise better means of distinguishing pre and post mortem wounds, but again, as in the ageing of injuries, these methods are still in the experimental stage.

The vital reactions described above take place in the soft tissues of the body. When dealing with skeletal remains, therefore, the distinc-tion between pre and post mortem wounds can often not be made.

3

DEATH
DUE TO NATURAL CAUSES

The largest single group of cases which comes to medico-legal investigation is that of sudden and unexplained death. Most will be found to have been instances of unsuspected or neglected disease. Many of these conditions present no problem either in diagnosis or in the recognition of their lethal role, but in others the causal relationships are less clear. No one above the age of 40 is entirely free from pathological changes and the distinction between the changes of "normal" ageing and those which might be regarded as "disease" is hazy and controversial. Furthermore, that someone had been suffering from a certain disease and had been expected to die from it, does not mean that, in fact, he did die from it. A patient in the terminal stages of an illness who had expressed the intention of altering his will, may well have met a sudden and premature end. Having found a possible cause of death, therefore, is not necessarily the same as having found the cause of death.

The simplest cases are those in which a lesion was found which had arisen shortly prior to death and which was incompatible with life, like a ruptured aorta, or one which, although not invariably fatal, often leads to sudden death, such as occlusion of a major coronary artery. Even then, questions may arise concerning the possible role of effort or emotion or of slight trauma in precipitating the final event, questions to which the pathologist can rarely give a definite answer.

More difficult are cases in which a condition was found which had clearly antedated death for a long time, such as narrowing of the coronary arteries. While the pathologist may have little doubt concerning the lethal nature of the condition, he is usually quite unable to explain why death occurred at a particular moment.

Of great importance in both a criminal and civil context, are cases of violent death in which disease was also found. Some very difficult questions are likely to arise. To what extent did such pre-existing disease predispose the victim to the injury? Did the disease process aggravate the effects of the injury or vice versa? Would the victim have survived the injury in the absence of disease? It lies in the nature of these questions that no definite answers are possible and that the opinion of the pathologist can, at best, be given in terms of probability.

When only minimal disease was found, the temptation to attribute great significance to the only finding in an otherwise uninformative autopsy is naturally great, but it is better to admit doubt and leave the case open than to label it with a spurious diagnosis. As will be shown in Chapter 15, there are common causes of death which leave no diagnostic findings at all.

The natural causes of sudden and unexpected death

In a modern industrial society diseases of the heart and blood vessels occupy undisputed first place amongst the causes of sudden death in previously apparently healthy adults. In the majority of these cases the coronary arteries are affected. Until recently it was believed that there had to be blockage of one of the arteries by a thrombus, but it is now known that only about half the cases show actual coronary thrombosis; the remainder show merely narrowing of the arteries of various degrees of severity. A part of the heart muscle may be found to have undergone local cellular breakdown because of lack of blood supply (heart infarct). Rarer cardiac causes of unexpected death include certain lesions of heart valves, especially insufficiency of the aortic valve, and inflammation of the heart muscle (myocarditis).

Next in frequency are conditions involving the brain and again disturbances of its blood supply are most common. A major artery may burst causing bleeding into the brain substance (intracerebral hemorrhage) or an artery may become blocked leading to local death of a part of the brain (brain infarct). Both conditions are popularly known as "stroke". A localized bulging (aneurysm) may develop in a weak spot in the wall of a brain artery and while this is usually clinically silent, rupture of such an aneurysm causes a massive hemorrhage either into the brain or into the space surrounding it (subarachnoid hemorrhage). Other brain lesions like abscesses or tumors are much rarer causes of unexpected exitus.

For a review of sudden death in young soldiers see Mortiz and Zamchek [124]* and in young adults Luke and Helpern.[103]

In children the spectrum of unexpectedly lethal disease is rather different. Heart and brain lesions are not nearly as prominent as in adults but infections, particularly of the respiratory system, play a much greater role. The condition known as "crib death", "cot death"

---

*References are to Bibliography beginning on page 159.

or "sudden infant death syndrome" (S.I.D.S.) to which infants 3 to 6 months of age succumb is discussed in Chapter 8.

Death due to fright. While folk lore abounds with stories of sudden death due to fright, usually in a voodoo setting, it seems doubtful whether this can occur in a normal individual. In previously damaged hearts, however, sudden emotional strain can induce serious functional disturbance [78, 160] and possibly death.

Status thymico-lymphaticus. This was at one time described as consisting of enlargement of the thymus and other lymphatic tissues of the body, often combined with unusually small adrenal glands and aorta. It is no longer accepted as a cause of sudden death [190] and the term is not in current scientific use.

Sickle cell crisis. This has only recently been recognized as a cause of sudden death in persons with Negro ancestry. The red blood cells, which contain an abnormal form of hemoglobin (hemoglobin S), become distorted when the oxygen tension falls and block small blood vessels throughout the body. This may occur during exertion, such as a fight, in an unpressurized aircraft or during surgical anaesthesia. The condition is not difficult to recognize at autopsy, provided the possibility of a sickle cell crisis is kept in mind.[109]

Anaphylaxis. This is an acute reaction caused by contact with an antigen, such as a drug or an insect sting, to which the person is unusually sensitive. It is thus not strictly due to "natural" causes but the initial insult may not have been witnessed. The findings are not diagnostic and usually include airway obstruction due to swelling of the lining of the larynx and edema of the lungs.

Sudden death in alcoholics. Sudden death is not infrequent in alcoholics and may not be due merely to an excessive alcohol intake or to aspiration of stomach contents. Many of these will be found to have large fatty livers but precisely what role this plays and whether fat embolism occurs is controversial.[44, 66, 107]

Iatrogenic disease. This group of disorders is, in some manner, caused by medical management and has also been called "diseases of medical progress". It grows larger and more varied as therapeutic and diagnostic procedures become more complex and aggressive. It includes mishaps during surgical operations, anaesthetic accidents, transfusions of incompatible blood, the administration of the wrong medication or the right medication in the wrong dosage, unusual reactions to drugs mostly to the antibiotics, local anaesthetics and radiological contrast media, and accidents during diagnostic procedures.

Included in this group are also such interesting and controversial problems as the tendency to thrombosis in women taking contraceptive medication and the liver damage which occasionally follows the administration of halothane anaesthetics.

For a review of iatrogenic disease see Moser.[125]

4

TRAFFIC FATALITIES.
"HIT AND RUN" ACCIDENTS

Mortality statistics provide an unconventional but informative insight into a society and its stage of technological development. As its population becomes more mobile and as it changes from an agricultural to a predominantly urban society, accidental deaths not only become more frequent but those due to the natural environment such as exposure, starvation and animal attacks are gradually replaced by those due to traffic and industrial mishaps and accidents in the home and during sport and recreation.

In most industrial nations motor vehicle accidents have become, by far, the predominant type of accidental death. In Canada in 1974, the last year for which complete data are avilable, 7.8 per cent of all deaths were accidental, an incidence of 57.7 per 100,000 population. The ten most common types of accidental death were motor vehicle (traffic) 48.1 per cent, falls 14.2 per cent, drowning 8.0 per cent, industrial type accidents 6.8 per cent, fire 6.1 per cent, poisonings 5.4 per cent, suffocation 4.3 per cent, aircraft accidents 1.3 per cent, firearms 0.9 per cent and motor vehicle (non-traffic) 0.8 per cent. The overall motor vehicle traffic fatality rate per 100,000 population was 27.7 and of all these traffic fatalities 82.1 per cent were due to injuries sustained in three types of accident, collision with another vehicle (40.7 per cent), loss of control (22.0 per cent) and collision with a pedestrian (19.5 per cent).[1*]

These figures do not reflect the full social and economic impact of traffic accidents because for each fatality many are injured and often permanently disabled. In Canada, in a typical year (1970), the ratio of dead to injured was 1 : 23.4 with property damage estimated at 311 million dollars.[129]

In most countries deaths in which a motor vehicle is known or suspected to have played a part become the subject of a medico-legal

*References are to Bibliography beginning on page 159.

investigation. Apart from drivers and their passengers, those examined include pedestrians, bicyclists, motorcyclists, road construction workers and children.

The pattern of injury

It is not surprising that a complex event like a traffic accident which involves many variables will produce a wide spectrum of injuries. In large scale studies, however, some patterns emerge. It is by the recognition of such patterns that forensic pathologists have contributed to safety by advocating such devices as seat belts, laminated glass, collapsible steering columns and improvements in highway design.

Pedestrians. A common type of fatal accident involves a single pedestrian and a single vehicle. A large variety of injuries may be produced and, unfortunately, their nomenclature is not uniform. Those sustained by the first contact with the vehicle are generally known as "primary impact" injuries, those sustained by being thrown on the hood or by being run over as "secondary impact" injuries and those incurred by falling on the road or by being dragged as "secondary" or "tertiary" injuries.

A pedestrian may receive a glancing impact from the side of a vehicle which causes a grazing injury to the body surface and which may rupture the liver, spleen or mesentery and which may throw him backwards inflicting secondary head injuries. Extensive lacerations of the subcutaneous tissues may be caused, especially in the regions of the hips and buttocks and in obese subjects. These may form large fluctuating pockets of macerated fat and blood, occasionally with only slight external signs of injury.

Impacts with the front of the vehicle, however, are more common. In an adult in the erect position the centre of gravity lies approximately at the level of the umbilicus. When struck by a passenger car, the primary impact is usually received well below the centre of gravity so that the body is thrown upwards, landing on the hood or the roof of the vehicle suffering secondary impact injuries to the head and upper limbs. A final fall on the pavement may inflict secondary injuries, particularly to the head, and these are often more lethal than the initial impact injuries.

The primary impact by the front of the vehicle often inflicts characteristic fractures of the lower legs ("bumper fractures") which are usually compound and often comminuted. The distance of these fractures from the heel is of obvious importance in indicating the height of the bumper, although as Spitz[166] points out, sudden braking will cause the front end of the car to dip and to lower the level of impact. Furthermore, if one leg was raised at the time, as in walking or running, it will have been struck at a lower level than the leg which had been in contact with the ground. Higher impacts frequently fracture the pelvic bone and the sacro-iliac joints.

In the case of adults struck by a larger vehicle, such as a truck, or in the case of children, the primary impact tends to be above the centre of gravity so that the body is thrown forwards and may be run over.

The injuries caused by wheels passing over a body are of two types. Their shearing effect, which is especially great when the wheels are locked, avulses the soft tissues and sometimes amputates limbs. Their weight may pulp the organs, crush the skull or chest and split the front of the pelvis, but in young children it is not uncommon to find extensive internal injuries without fractures. The details of tire marks (Fig. 4-2) may become very important when the responsible vehicle has not been apprehended.

When the body has been dragged, its surface may be extensively abraded and contain embedded sand or gravel. The friction on the road surface may have created sufficient heat to have caused actual thermal burns.

Cyclists and motorcyclists. Again, the relation of the primary impact to the centre of gravity determines the direction in which the body is thrown. Head injuries are very common but the protective value of helmets is still controversial. Campbell [25] found helmets to give a significant degree of protection but this view is not shared by Ryan.[152]

Car occupants. A moving car may collide with another moving vehicle or with a stationary object, roll over or be subjected to a combination of these events. In any case, its sudden deceleration or change of direction will cause its occupants to be thrown against its interior. In a rolling or spinning vehicle the doors may open and the occupants may be ejected. Many kinds of injury may be sustained.

In head-on collisions the front end of the vehicle suffers the primary impact and, by being crushed, absorbs the shock of the collision. The car occupants, however, keep on moving forwards and, if not restrained, strike the relatively unyielding objects of the front interior (Fig. 4-1). Even in a head-on collision of only 30 miles per hour the occupants strike the interior with a kinetic energy of several thousand pounds. In a recent study[188] 30 per cent of fatal injuries were caused by the steering wheel assembly, 22 percent by the surface of the car's interior, 30 per cent by the exterior of the car or by being thrown out of the car, 20 per cent by the windshield frame, 12 per cent by the roof, 11 per cent by the instrument panel and 8 per cent by the windshield. (These percentages add up to more than 100 because some occupants sustained fatal injuries from more than one object.)

In such head-on collisions the knees of the front seat occupants

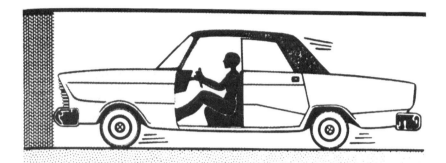

0.000 seconds - car hits barrier

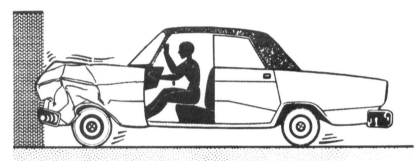

0.100 seconds - car stops

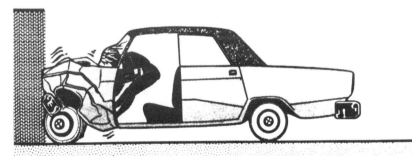

0.120 seconds - person hits car interior

Fig. 4-1. In front end collisions the vehicle sustains the primary impact and this is followed by the secondary impact of the occupants against the car's interior. [Courtesy, Ministry of Transportation and Communications, Province of Ontario.]

come into forceful contact with the lower edge of the dashboard and sustain fractures of the knee cap and lower end of the thighbone and, by transmitted force, fractures and dislocations of the hip.[68] The chest of the driver may strike the steering wheel and suffer rib fractures and fractures of the breast bone (sternum) resulting in the clinical picture of the "floating" or "flail" chest. This "steering wheel" injury may also include rupture of the heart chambers and aorta and lacerations of the liver.

Late clinical complications of such blunt impacts to the chest are gradually being recognized. These include contusions of the heart[10, 73] and lungs and injuries of the aorta which may eventually lead to aneurysms.

Fractures and fracture-dislocations of the ankles are common in front seat occupants and these are caused either by direct force while the feet are resting on the floor boards or by being wedged or twisted under the front seats. Unrestrained back seat occupants may be catapulted forwards inflicting head and neck injuries on the front seat occupants.

All individuals subjected to sudden deceleration may incur inertial injury of the aorta which usually takes the form of transverse tears. If the tear involves all layers of the vessel wall a rapidly fatal hemorrhage will ensue. If the tear is incomplete, the area will constitute a weak spot on which an aneurysm may develop after months or years.

The effects of seat belts

The value of seat belts in the avoidance of injury is no longer questioned. They prevent ejection from the car and impact against its interior. By prolonging the "stopping distance" and by distributing the impact over a large area they reduce the kinetic force acting on the body. The fact that seat belts themselves may be instrumental in causing injury is not so widely known.

Sudden deceleration will cause forward flexion across a lap type seat belt and impact of the head or face against the dashboard or the back of the front seat. The main value of the diagonal type of belt lies in preventing this type of injury.

Of more importance because of the greater difficulty of recognition are internal injuries which may lead to death several hours after the accident. These include tears of the mesentery and intestine, ruptures of the liver, spleen, pancreas and common bile duct, rupture of the gravid uterus and of major blood vessels. While, again, the lap type belt seems to be the most hazardous, these injuries have also been reported in passengers wearing the diagonal type of belt.[74]

The mechanism whereby seat belts cause injury is complex. Direct crushing of the abdominal organs between the belt and the spine probably accounts for the injuries to the liver and spleen, especially if a lap type belt has been worn improperly, i.e. across the abdomen rather than across the pelvis. In very sudden deceleration at high speed jack-knifing across the belt may cause fractures of the lower spine. It is also likely that the inertia of fluid filled organs, such as loops of intestine and blood vessels, produces a shearing effect which injures these structures.[6, 170]

For discussions concerning the merits of the various types of seat belt see Lister and Milson,[100] Hebert[80] and Birrell.[19]

The role of disease or intoxication

Whether disease or intoxication played a part in the causation of an accident must be asked with regard to the drivers as well as pedestrians. It seems obvious at first sight that sudden illness on the part of the driver must be a frequent cause of accidents and there are, in fact, many statistics to support this view. Peterson and Petty [134] found that 19 per cent of drivers who died following an accident brought about by their own fault, died of disease, mostly of a cardiovascular nature, and not of trauma.

However, like so many conclusions which seemed obvious at first sight, the premises upon which they were based may not have been true. Other studies have found that acute illness played only a minor role in the causation of accidents.[67] There are probably very few medical catastrophes which would not allow a driver the few seconds needed to bring the vehicle to a stop or at least to slow it down sufficiently to prevent a major accident. Baker and Spitz [7] make the interesting suggestion that the high prevalence of arteriosclerotic heart disease in fatally injured drivers did not reflect a causal relationship but merely the greater tendency of the older drivers to succumb to their injuries. Most countries have rather stringent laws concerning the issue of driving licences to persons with a history of epilepsy, but epilepsy has been found to play a part in only a very few accidents.[47]

In the case of pedestrians, many of which are in the higher age groups, the question of a seeing or hearing disability arises. While this makes it obligatory to examine the eyes and ears, it must be admitted that their function cannot usually be assessed on the basis of post mortem findings.

There is an uncommon but encouraging unanimity amongst investigators concerning the role which alcohol plays in traffic accidents. It is, without doubt, the most important single contributing factor. In a Canadian study of 2,481 drivers who died within 6 hours after the accident 1,378 (55.5 per cent) had a positive blood alcohol, while of 572 pedestrians who died within 6 hours 306 (53.5 per cent) were to some extent intoxicated.[26] For a review of the effects of alcohol on driving ability see Smith.[163a]

The magnitude of the problem created by other drugs, particularly the tranquillizers, sedatives, narcotics, antihistamines and stimulants is less well defined but is sufficiently great to require a toxicological analysis in all cases in which the history of the deceased, his personal effects or the circumstances of the accident make it seem possible that these drugs may have played a part. On the other hand, screening all cases for these drugs will give only a meagre return for the large amount of work involved.

Who was the driver?

The original location of the various occupants of the vehicle must be deduced from the locations in which they were found, from the distribution of blood stains within the vehicle and from the nature of their injuries, including imprints of dashboard knobs, and the typical "steering wheel" injury of the chest and abdomen of the driver. Imprints of the pattern on the accelerator and brake pedals have been found on the soles of the driver's shoes.[86]

"Hit and run" accidents

The discovery of a body on or near a highway immediately raises the suspicion that death may have resulted from an unwitnessed ("hit and run") accident, especially if it bears marks or injuries which could be attributed to a motor vehicle. In addition to the usual problem of identity, the questions which arise and in which the pathologist will be asked to give some guidance to the investigating officers include the following:

(1) Had the deceased in fact been struck by a vehicle?
(2) What type of vehicle was involved?
(3) What were the relative positions of vehicle and victim?
(4) Could the deceased have been struck by more than one vehicle?
(5) Could the deceased have been lying on the ground when struck?
(6) Could the injuries have been sustained after death?
(7) Did the accident occur where the body was found?

These cases make great demands upon the examiner although not all of the above questions can be answered on the basis of the medical findings alone. The pathologist usually works under pressure and in conditions less than ideal but his findings are important in the reconstruction of events and give direction to the early stages of the search for the responsible vehicle. He must, therefore, be given all information before the autopsy and, if at all possible, an opportunity of visiting the scene.

In no other case is the pathologist so directly concerned with the collection of trace evidence. The following steps are recommended when examining victims of "hit and run" accidents.

The clothing is inspected for fragments of glass, paint or chromium

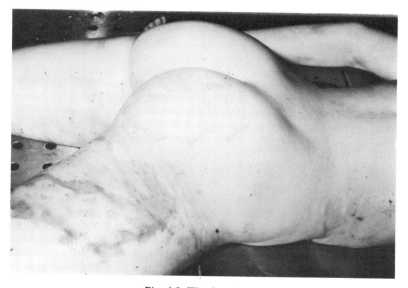

Fig. 4-2. Tire imprints.

and each item of clothing is put into a separate plastic container. Clothing must not be shaken or allowed to fall on the floor.

Each external wound is described in detail, photographed (with scale) and its distance from the nearest heel measured.

All wounds are searched for sand, gravel, glass fragments or paint chips.

The body surface is inspected for imprints of headlights, bumpers, hood ornaments etc. and for tire marks, remembering that all these may become more distinct after the first 24 hours (Fig. 4-3). Both imprints and tire marks must be measured and photographed in situ, as removal and fixation causes distortion. Spitz [166] recommends the use of transparent parchment paper as a permanent record.

X-rays of the body show not only metallic foreign bodies but also the distribution of bone fragments which, in turn, may indicate the direction of impacts. The distance of all fractures from the nearest heel is also measured.

In addition to taking specimens for toxicological analysis, the pathologist must obtain samples of scalp hair and of blood for blood group determination.

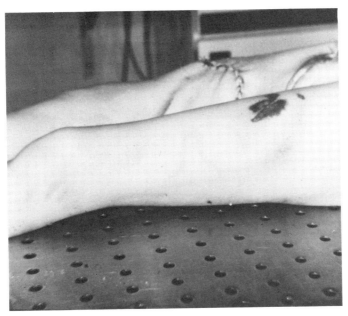

Fig. 4-3. This impression of the car bumper did not become visible on the skin until 24 hours after the autopsy.

5

POISONINGS
AND INTOXICATIONS

Poisoning, from the forensic viewpoint, is the presence in the body of any noxious substance which, directly or indirectly, caused death. The presence of substances which played a mere contributory role is usually designated by the term "intoxication". That this distinction is arbitrary and that the precise role of a toxic agent in a given case may be difficult to assess is obvious.

As poisoning or intoxication may be caused by all licit or illicit medicinal preparations, all industrial and household chemicals, the products of combustion, animal and insect venoms and bacterial and plant toxins, the number of substances which may be involved is almost infinite. The variety of toxic agents encountered in actual practice, however, is relatively small and reflects their use and availability in the community, changing gradually as new products appear on the market and the use of others is abandoned.

The clinical course of poisoning may range from a rapid, almost instantaneous, demise to a prolonged illness caused by the slow accumulation of a toxic substance. Of particular interest and forensic importance are those instances in which the victim survives the immediate effects of the poison only to succumb, after a period of apparent recovery, to its delayed effects. Examples of such a course of events may be found in poisonings by carbon monoxide, phosphorus, organic solvents and ethylene glycol ("anti-freeze").

Homicidal poisoning, which has a long and colourful history, has become much rarer in modern times, partly because of the uncertainty of results and partly because of the greater chance of detection. The majority of fatal poisonings encountered nowadays in adults are suicidal while those in children are accidental.

Poisons may act by local irritation or systemically. A few substances, such as phenol, have both a local destructive as well as a systemic toxic effect.

The clinical signs and symptoms of most forms of poisoning are indistinguishable from those of natural disease, so that the pathologist must always keep in mind the possibility of poisoning and must be informed of the circumstances under which death appeared to have occurred. Not only must he be told of the finding of pills, syringes, drinking glasses, plastic bags, hypodermic needles and eye droppers at the scene but he must also receive all available information concerning the medical background of the deceased, his occupation, any medication taken, any history of drug abuse and the course of the final illness. If the pathologist does not possess this information he will start his investigation at a disadvantage and instances of poisoning may be missed.

Few post mortem findings are sufficiently characteristic to indicate poisoning by a specific agent. Many fatal poisonings cannot be recognized or even suspected on the basis of post mortem findings and the pathologist must rely on the chemical analysis of tissues and body fluids. To the alert observer, however, some post mortem appearances may suggest the presence of certain toxic substances. The list given below is not complete but does include the more commonly encountered poisons.

Corrosion of lips, mouth and stomach	Strong acids and alkalis, phenol, fluorides.
Odour	Formaldehyde, cyanides, methyl salicylate ("Oil of Wintergreen"), paraldehyde, acetone, carbon tetrachloride, ammonia, naphthalene (moth repellent), camphor, phenol, ether, chloroform.
Change in the colour of lividity	Bright pink — carbon monoxide, brown — nitrites, nitrates, nitrobenzene, aniline, bromates, chlorates, hydrogen sulphide.
Thrombosed superficial veins, needle marks	Narcotics, amphetamines.
Skin blisters	Barbiturates, carbon monoxide.
Fatty, swollen liver	Alcohol, phosphorus, carbon tetrachloride, arsenic, toluene, naphthalene, chloroform.
Pale, swollen kidneys	Mercury bichloride, carbon tetrachloride, ethylene glycol, bromates, oxalates.
Hemorrhages	Benzene, warfarin, salicylates, snake venom.
Hemolysis	Tap water (intravenously), naphthalene.

The role of the pathologist in cases of suspected poisoning or drug overdose

The pathologist is responsible for taking appropriate specimens for analysis during the autopsy, for their packaging and labelling, for their storage and conveyance to the laboratory. In court he can be expected to testify concerning the structural changes in tissues caused by toxic substances but, unless he possesses expertise beyond his own specialty, he would not be qualified to give evidence concerning the pharmacological effects of toxic agents, their chemical structure or the analytic techniques employed.

There is generally no need to modify the ordinary autopsy procedure in cases of suspected poisoning or drug overdose apart from the steps involved in securing the samples for analysis. The body surface is inspected for indications of drug addiction such as needle marks or skin abscesses and the mouth, rectum and vagina are examined for concealed drugs. Internal findings like inflammation of the liver or lymph nodes or an enlarged spleen may also suggest drug abuse.

As in the interpretation of toxicological findings the possibility, albeit remote, of accidental contamination of the specimens or their mislabelling must always be considered, the pathologist should be questioned concerning the manner in which the specimens were obtained.

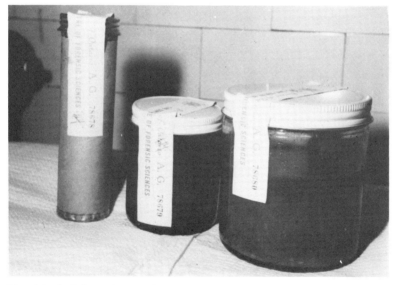

Fig. 5-1. Sealed specimens of blood and stomach contents for toxicological analysis.

(1) The body should not be washed prior to autopsy. Any powdery or crystalline deposits on the skin should be removed and collected in a dry container.

(2) No disinfectant or deodorant solutions should be sprayed into the air of the room or applied to the body.

(3) Smoking must not be permitted near the autopsy table.

(4) Clean, preferably new, glass jars with tightly fitting screw

tops should be used to hold the specimens. If the containers are not new, they should be thoroughly rinsed with tap water and a sample of the tap water submitted.

(5) Each specimen should be put into a separate container.

(6) No preservative or fixative should be added except to the blood sample for alcohol determination.

(7) The gastro-intestinal tract should be opened only after all other samples have been taken and sealed.

(8) Specimens accidentally dropped on the floor must be discarded.

(9) The containers should be sealed in such a way that they could not be opened without breaking the seal. The seals should bear an identifying number and be intialled by the pathologist (Fig. 5-1).

(10) The specimens should be refrigerated or frozen until their submission to the laboratory.

Specimens to be taken for a General Poison Screen:

(1) 10 millilitres of blood with preservative (sodium fluoride) for alcohol determination,

(2) 200 millilitres of blood without preservative,

(3) all stomach contents,

(4) all urine,

(5) 500 grams of liver.

Additional specimens to be taken when certain poisons are suspected:

Arsenic

A bundle of scalp hair, two complete fingernails, the entire intestine (tied in segments), one kidney, 60 grams of bone.

Heavy metals (lead, mercury, bismuth)

One kidney, contents of large intestine, 60 grams of bone. (Metal containers must not be used.)

Alkaloids (narcotics, atropine, strychnine)

500 millilitres of blood without preservative, bile, if needle marks are present, the entire needle track with 2 centimetres of surrounding tissue.

Volatile poisons (kerosene, ether, chloroform, benzine)

One half of each lung, 500 grams of brain tissue (plastic bags must not be used as containers).

Cyanides

500 grams of brain tissue.

All suspect containers like cups, glasses, bottles and syringes found at the scene should also be submitted to the laboratory, as well as all powders, medicinal preparations or prescriptions found at the scene or in pockets.

The significance of drugs or poisons found post mortem

In order to establish the lethal role of a given drug or poison, it should ideally be shown that the particular agent had been introduced into the body in sufficient quantity to have caused death, that the terminal illness and the post mortem findings were compatible with poisoning by the agent and that there was no other cause of death. These classical postulates cannot be fulfilled in every case because:

(1) Toxic agents may kill by mechanisms other than by excessive dosage, namely by hypersensitivity reactions or by the less well understood phenomenon generally known as "idiosyncrasy".

(2) Drugs may potentiate each other. This applies particularly to depressants of the nervous system such as alcohol and barbiturates. Their combined effect may be lethal although neither may be present in excessive amount.

(3) There are great differences in susceptibility or, conversely, in tolerance, to drugs and poisons between individuals, so that it is generally not possible to speak of "lethal doses" or "lethal blood levels" but merely of "lethal ranges".

(4) Pre-existing disease may make an individual especially susceptible. For example, heart disease, in which the blood supply to the heart is precarious, will predispose a person to the effects of agents which interfere with the oxygen transport of the circulation, such as carbon monoxide.

(5) An individual may sustain lethal damage by a toxic substance but survive long enough to eliminate much or all of it, so that at the time of the post mortem examination it may not be present in large amounts or may not be demonstrable at all.

Until the early part of this century it was possible for the pathologist to possess a comprehensive knowledge of the chemical and pharmacological properties of most poisons and medicinal preparations. The number and variety of noxious substances to which an individual may be exposed in a modern environment is now so great that the fields of industrial and pharmaceutical toxicology are no longer regarded as being within the scope of pathology and such evidence is now generally given by experts in these disciplines. Nevertheless, a few toxic agents, such as alcohol, carbon monoxide and the barbiturates, are of such wide occurrence that the pathologist can be expected to be, to some extent, familiar with them.

Some of the questions which commonly arise in court are briefly discussed below. For details and for information concerning other toxic substances textbooks of forensic medicine and toxicology should be consulted.

ETHYL ALCOHOL

The consumption of alcoholic beverages is such a firmly established part of our culture that ethyl alcohol is by far the most commonly encountered toxic agent in forensic work. Death due to ethyl alcohol per se is rare but its role in contributing to accidents, altercations and many forms of delinquent behaviour is too well known to require further discussion. Furthermore, some conditions, such as the impaction of a food bolus in the larynx or death from exposure in an urban environment, rarely occur in the absence of alcohol.

It is not feasible to examine every autopsy case for the presence of alcohol without placing an excessive burden on the laboratory. Apart from the instances mentioned above, an analysis for alcohol should be done in all traffic fatalities (drivers and pedestrians), all deaths occurring in fires and following industrial accidents, deaths resulting from fights and in all obscure deaths.

A survival time of more than 24 hours will usually permit the metabolism and elimination of alcohol and thus make an analysis unrewarding.

The alcohol content of common beverages

The alcohol content of beverages is expressed as the percentage of absolute alcohol by volume.

Beer, ale, stout	2 - 6 %
Wines (dry, unfortified), e.g. claret, Rhine wines, sparkling wines, rosé	10 - 15 %
Wines (sweet, fortified), e.g. sherry, port, madeira, malaga, muscatel	10 - 14 %
Cider	8 - 12 %
Liqueurs	30 - 45 %
Spirits, e.g. brandy, whisky, bourbon, rum, gin, vodka	40 - 45 %

The strength of spirits is usually designated by "proof". The defiinition of this standard in Britain and Canada is different from that in the United States of America. See Table 5-2.

Table 5-2

Liquor Strength Conversion Chart

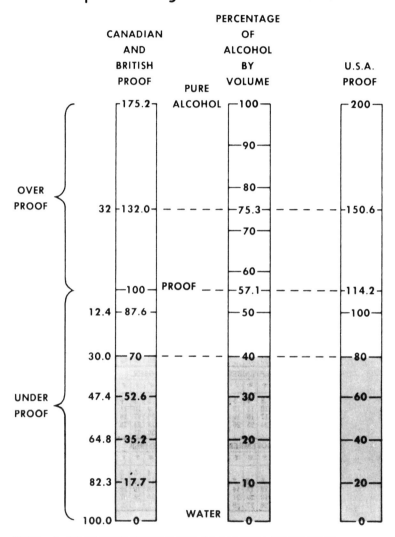

NOTE: 1. START WITH PERCENTAGE OF ALCOHOL BY VOLUME

2. TO CONVERT TO CANADIAN PROOF MULTIPLY IT BY 1.75

3. TO CONVERT TO U.S.A. PROOF MULTIPLY IT BY 2

Reproduced by permission of The Liquor Control Board of Ontario.

The absorption of alcohol and its distribution in the body

Alcohol is quickly absorbed from the empty stomach and from the intestine. Following a single drink, alcohol is detectable in the blood within 5 minutes, reaches the maximum blood level in 30 to 40 minutes and is completely absorbed within 2 hours. Food in the stomach and dilution of the alcohol will prolong absorption and reduce the maximum blood level.

During the absorptive phase the alcohol content of the cerebrospinal fluid and of the organs lags behind that of the blood while in the post-absorptive phase it is higher.[105]* Only in the relatively brief period of equilibrium does the alcohol level of the blood reflect the alcohol content of the tissues.

In this period of equilibrium the differences in alcohol content between the various organs are slight. The brain shows the most consistent relationship to the blood level and, being relatively resistant to putrefaction, is the most suitable organ for analysis in decomposing bodies. Next in suitability appears to be skeletal muscle.

Table 5-3

Blood level of alcohol			Clinical manifestations**
Percentage	Grams per litre, parts per thousand (0/00)	Milligrams per decilitre (mg%, mg/dl)	
0.005	0.05	5	
0.01	0.1	10	Normal by ordinary observation
0.02	0.2	20	
0.03	0.3	30	
0.04	0.4	40	Decreased inhibitions (loquaciousness,
0.05	0.5	50	jocularity, aggressiveness).
0.06	0.6	60	Some impairment in the performance
0.07	0.7	70	of skilled tasks.
0.08	0.8	80	COMMON STATUTORY DRIVING LIMIT
0.09	0.9	90	Incoordination of fine muscular
0.10	1.0	100	movements, slurring of speech.
0.12	1.2	120	Decreased response to stimuli
0.14	1.4	140	(loss of protective reflexes).
0.16	1.6	160	Decreased pain sensation.
0.18	1.8	180	
0.20	2.0	200	Staggering gait, blurred vision,
0.25	2.5	250	loss of balance.
0.30	3.0	300	Coma, hypothermia.
0.35	3.5	350	
0.40	4.0	400	Beginning of lethal range.
0.45	4.5	450	

*References are to the Bibliography beginning on page 159.

**These apply to the absorptive phase and show considerable variation between individuals. In the post-absorptive phase clinical recovery tends to be more rapid than the fall in the blood alcohol level.

Alcohol consumption and body alcohol content

How much alcohol would have to be consumed in order to attain this blood level? This question which recurs in court can rarely be answered with certainty because the height of the blood level depends not only on the amount of alcohol consumed but also on the length of time during which drinking took place. Thus the consumption of a given amount of alcohol over a short period would raise the blood level higher than the consumption of the same amount over a longer period. The interval between the last drink and death often introduces further uncertainty.

The best that can usually be accomplished is an estimate of the amount of alcohol in the body at the time of examination by employing Widmark's equation

$$A = p \times c \times r$$

where A = total weight of alcohol in grams absorbed by the body

p = weight of subject in kilograms

c = milligrams of alcohol per gram of whole blood

r = ratio of alcohol absorbed by unit weight of body to alcohol absorbed by unit weight of whole blood (0.68 for men, 0.55 for women).

A "drink" is usually defined as 1½ fluid ounces (42.6 millilitres) of 40 per cent whisky, gin, rum or vodka and is equivalent to 12 fluid ounces (341 millilitres) of beer or one 5 fluid ounce (142 millilitre) glass of wine or champagne.

It is clear that the consumption must always have been greater than the body alcohol content, but by how much depends on the variables mentioned above.

Elimination and rate of disappearance

About 90 per cent of the ingested alcohol is oxidized, mostly in the liver, the remainder being excreted in the urine, sweat and in the expired air.

The rate of disappearance is about 15 milligrams per 100 millilitres of blood per hour or 100 milligrams per kilogram of body weight per hour, but there may be considerable differences between individuals. Exercise, drugs, vitamins or eating do not seem to affect the rate of elimination,[29] nor does sleep or unconsciousness,[142] but advanced liver disease may retard its oxidation.

The effect of vomiting is complex and depends on the time of vomiting in relation to the time of drinking and its severity. While tending to evacuate the unabsorbed alcohol from the stomach and thus retard the rise in the blood level, the increased intestinal activity and congestion associated with vomiting leads to a more rapid absorption from the intestinal lumen. Thus no correction need generally be applied to account for vomiting,[142] although it may influence the measurement of alcohol in breath (see below).

A survival period of several hours following an injury may permit a reduction or even disappearance of the alcohol in the circulating blood. If the injury resulted in internal bleeding and the collection of blood in a body cavity (hematoma), the alcohol in such a hematoma would persist much longer and would reflect the blood alcohol level at the time of injury better than the peripheral blood.[84]

Alcohol in the urine

The alcohol content of the urine should be determined whenever possible because it may help in the evaluation of the blood alcohol level. It is also less altered by putrefaction, so that the presence of alcohol in the urine of a decomposing body is of greater significance than its presence in the blood (see below). For practical purposes post mortem diffusion of alcohol in and out of the urinary bladder does not occur.[186] Again, in the case of long survivals the alcohol content of the urine may be more informative than the blood alcohol level.[5]

In contrast to the situation in the living subject, the interpretation of the post mortem urinary findings is relatively simple. The alcohol level of the urine which is being excreted bears the ratio of about 1.33 : 1 to that of the blood (urine alcohol x 0.7 = blood alcohol). [43, 82, 132] The urine in the bladder, on the other hand, has collected since the last micturition and its alcohol level, therefore, reflects merely the average blood level during that period. The shorter this period is, the closer is the agreement between the average blood level calculated on the basis of the urinary findings and the actual blood alcohol level.

If the blood alcohol level, as calculated on the basis of the urinary alcohol level, is higher than the actual blood level found at autopsy, the blood alcohol level was in the process of falling, conversely if the calculated blood level is lower than that found, the individual was still in the absorptive phase.

Alcohol in breath

The technical difficulties and legal problems involved in obtaining blood samples for analysis have led to the introduction of several instruments which measure the alcohol level in expired air. These include the "Breathalyzer" developed by Borkenstein in 1954.

The blood circulating through the vast network of capillary blood vessels in the lungs is separated from the air in the air sacs (alveoli) only by a delicate membrane. Alcohol, therefore, rapidly diffuses from the blood into the alveolar air, quickly reaching an equilibrium, so that 2,100 millilitres of alveolar air contain the same amount of alcohol as 1 millilitre of blood at 31°C (the usual temperature of expired air). The various instruments are usually calibrated in such a way that the blood alcohol level can be read directly.

While generally the readings accurately reflect the blood alcohol level, several possible sources of error must be kept in mind, apart from any malfunctioning or improper calibration of the instrument itself. As indicated above, it is the air from the deepest parts of the respiratory system which is in equilibrium with the blood alcohol, so that a deep expiration into the instrument is required for an accurate reading. A shallow expiration, consisting largely of air from the mouth and windpipe, will give a misleading result. Any alcohol in the mouth as the result of recent drinking, vomiting or the use of alcoholic mouth washes, will introduce a significant error, so that no readings should be taken within 15 minutes of these events.

Can significant amounts of alcohol be absorbed by inhalation?

As might be expected, alcohol which readily diffuses from the blood into the air can also diffuse in the opposite direction. Whether significant blood alcohol levels could be acquired in this way, by breathing air containing alcohol vapour, is still unsettled. Mason[113] found no absorption in adult subjects under experimental conditions but a newborn infant who was accidentally exposed to alcohol vapour acquired a lethal blood concentration.[57]

Post mortem stability

Under conditions of normal refrigeration no significant change in the alcohol content of the body occurs until putrefaction supervenes, although diffusion from the stomach may take place (see below).

Post mortem diffusion of alcohol

Diffusion of alcohol may occur after death through the stomach wall into the chest cavities and into the fluid in the pericardial sac.[81, 139, 140] Although very little penetrates into the chambers of the heart, contamination of heart blood by the pericardial fluid during the collection of the blood sample may introduce considerable error. It is, therefore, better to obtain the blood sample from one of the peripheral veins before the opening of the chest.

The effects of putrefaction

Putrefaction, which involves the fermentation of carbohydrates by bacterial and yeast ferments, results in the transient appearance of ethyl alcohol in the tissues. This has been demonstrated in cadavers[61, 150] as well as in blood putrefying in vitro.[20] This production of alcohol is especially pronounced in the brain and liver of submerged bodies so that these organs should not be taken for analysis in such cases.[61] At the same time, alcohol is broken down, slowly under refrigeration but quite rapidly at room temperature, so that in a putrefying cadaver there may be simultaneous formation and oxidation of alcohol.

The level of alcohol generated during putrefaction does not usually exceed 20 milligrams per decilitre so that levels above this indicate consumption. The degree of intoxication however, cannot be assessed in decomposing bodies.

The formation of alcohol in vitro

That ethyl alcohol can be formed in vitro during storage or transit has now been established. Concentrations of a preservative such as sodium fluoride which may be adequate to prevent bacterial growth may not inhibit the growth of yeasts.[64, 140]

In order to reduce the chance of contamination the blood specimen should be obtained early in the course of the autopsy before the respiratory and intestinal tracts have been opened. The samples should be firmly stoppered and refrigerated.

In case of doubt it may be necessary to ascertain the sterility of the specimen. Any organisms grown on culture should be tested for their ability to produce alcohol in a sugar containing medium.

The effect of heat

There is no reason to believe that alcohol is generated during exposure to heat, so that the finding of alcohol in a burned body indicates consumption. The theoretical possibility that alcohol may be lost by evaporation has not been supported experimentally.[11]

The effect of skin preparation

In living subjects 70 per cent alcohol or alcoholic antiseptic solutions are commonly employed in the cleaning of the skin prior to venepuncture. While these should obviously be avoided when blood samples for alcohol determination are being taken, it seems that any contamination of the blood sample which might occur is minimal. On the other hand, needles and syringes which have been kept in alcohol and incompletely dried can cause significant error. Methods of collecting blood samples at autopsy do not usually involve the use of needles or syringes or skin preparation.

Alcohol in the embalmed body

The process of embalming includes the perfusion of the body with fluids which may contain ethyl or methyl alcohol and the draining of the blood. The significance of either the presence or the absence of alcohol in an embalmed body is therefore uncertain. See also Chapter 14.

Is there a "normal" blood alcohol level?

The intestine of the normal individual always contains bacteria and yeasts capable of fermenting carbohydrates and it is not unreasonable to expect that alcohol might be produced and be detectable in the blood stream during abstinence from alcoholic beverages. Traces have, in fact, been reported by several investigators. There is some doubt whether all of this "apparent alcohol" is ethyl alcohol and, in any event, no levels higher than 4 milligrams per 100 millilitres have been reported.[163]

Summary of sources of error

The blood level of alcohol found in a post mortem blood sample may be spuriously low because of breakdown during putrefaction or a long survival time or spuriously high because of production during putrefaction, fermentation in vitro or diffusion from the stomach. The action of alcohol may also have been potentiated by nervous depressants like the barbiturates or the tranquilizers.

CARBON MONOXIDE

Carbon monoxide is the product of the incomplete combustion of organic materials. It is formed in fires, especially of the smoldering type, and is a major constituent of coal gas and motor exhaust fumes. While natural gas does not normally contain carbon monoxide, its incomplete combustion in faulty appliances can quickly evolve lethal concentrations.

Carbon monoxide produces rapid anoxia by forming a relatively stable combination with hemoglobin (carboxyhemoglobin). This not only displaces oxygen from the blood but impairs the elimination of carbon dioxide.

Deaths due to carbon monoxide inhalation are still seen frequently, the gradual replacement of coal gas by natural gas and electricity being largely compensated by the ever increasing use of motor vehicles and small gasoline engines.

The inhalation of carbon monoxide will quickly establish toxic blood levels, their height depending on the concentration in the air, the period of exposure and the physical activity of the individual (Fig. 5-4).

"Normal" blood levels

Smokers and those exposed to heavy traffic may "normally" show some carboxyhemoglobin. Gettler and Mattice[56] found levels of 0.1 to 4.1 per cent in 18 persons living in New York City under conditions of minimal exposure. Twelve street cleaners, mostly smokers, showed saturations of 1.2 to 6.9 per cent. Blood saturations above 10 per cent generally indicate an "abnormal" exposure.

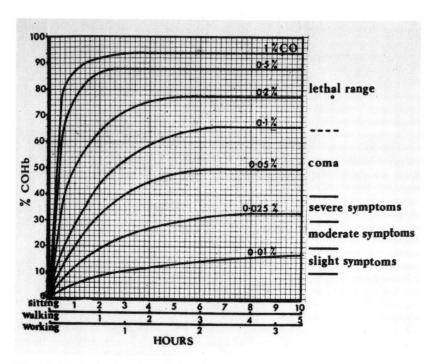

Fig. 5-4. Graph showing the relation of the carbon monoxide content of the blood to the carbon monoxide concentration in the air, the time of exposure and the type of activity. Modified from May,[114] by permission of the Editors, Archiv f. Gewebepath. u. Gewerbehyg.

Lethal blood levels

These show great individual variation. It appears that a slow rise in carbon monoxide saturation is better tolerated than a rapid accumulation.

In 304 cases Cimbura and co-workers found a range of lethal

concentrations from 23 to 89 per cent with a mean value of 51.4 per cent. They found that alcohol or barbiturates did not enhance the toxicity of carbon monoxide but that concomitant heart or respiratory disease lowered the mean lethal blood level to 46.2 per cent.[31]

Post mortem findings

The well known bright red lividity appears whenever the carbon monoxide saturation of the blood approaches 20 per cent. It is indistinguishable from that produced by cold, but in carbon monoxide poisoning this bright red colour will be found in the muscles and internal organs as well as on the body surface. Levels of carbon monoxide saturation below 20 per cent may not show the typical appearance.

Blisters of the skin, particularly at pressure points such as heels and elbows are occasionally found. These break easily exposing the deeper layers of the skin.

Otherwise the findings are not characteristic. In victims of fire the effects of heat are often superimposed on those of carbon monoxide poisoning and may occasionally obscure these. See Chapter 7.

Microscopically the pathological alterations are confined to the brain and depend on the length of survival. They are essentially those of lack of oxygen (anoxia). In long survivals lesions in a certain part of the brain (globus pallidus) have been described as well as a loss of white matter.[32, 33, 62]

Carbon monoxide and post mortem changes

There is nothing to suggest that carbon monoxide in the body modifies the progress of post mortem changes or that, conversely, putrefaction affects carbon monoxide levels,[42] although Curry believes that small amounts of carbon monoxide may be evolved after death.[35]

Post mortem stability

Carboxyhemoglobin is notoriously stable, especially in the absence of oxygen. It has been demonstrated on many occasions after long periods of burial.[75, 136]

For a discussion of carbon monoxide in victims of fire see Chapter 7.

BARBITURATES

The barbiturates derivatives of barbituric acid, are depressants of the central nervous system and are employed as hypnotics, sedatives and anticonvulsants. The nature of their chemical side chains determines the rapidity and duration of their action. The long acting group includes barbital and phenobarbital, the intermediate group amobarbital and the short acting group pentobarbital and secobarbital. An ultra short acting group, which includes thiopental, is used for intravenous anaesthesia but is rarely encountered in forensic work.

Dosage and blood levels

Hypnotic doses range from 0.1 to 0.3 grams. Therapeutic blood levels are usually less than 0.5 milligrams per 100 millilitres of blood in the case of the short and intermediate acting compounds but chronic users of phenobarbital, such as epileptics, may show levels of 5 milligrams per 100 millilitres. Lethal levels are very variable. Generally, in the case of the long acting group the lethal range is above 10 milligrams, in the intermediate group above 7 milligrams and in the short acting group above 3 milligrams. Other nervous system depressants, like alcohol, potentiate the effects of the barbiturates and lower the lethal ranges.[31, 88, 146]

Distribution in the body

Barbiturates are readily absorbed from all parts of the digestive tract, diffused throughout the tissues and across the placenta. They are evenly distributed through the nervous system[115] and reach their highest concentration in the liver.[172] The ultra short acting group is concentrated in the fatty tissues.[147]

Fate

The long and intermediate acting compounds are largely excreted in the urine while the short and ultra short acting barbiturates are metabolized in the liver. In toxic doses all compounds are excreted in the urine.[185]

Effects of overdosage

There is a general depression of brain activity which may result in temporary silence in the electroencephalogram. Occasionally elevation of mood (euphoria) and excitement are produced. In high doses there appears to be a direct depression of the heart muscle.

Autopsy findings

These are not diagnostic. Blisters of the skin may be present but these are not specific.[16, 176] Pneumonia is a common terminal event. In acute poisoning irreversible brain damage may be produced but survival may be sufficiently long to permit the drug to be eliminated before death.

Post mortem persistence

Barbiturates are very stable. They have been detected in formalin fixed tissue,[172] in liver fixed in embalming fluid[4] and during putrefaction.[4]

6

DEATH IN THE WATER

Few examinations are as demanding as those of bodies recovered from water or washed ashore. In addition to the cause of death, questions of identity and the time and place of death may arise, often made more difficult by post mortem changes and a large variety of post mortem artefacts. Not all individuals found under these circumstances met their death in the water and not all who did, drowned.

Did death occur in the water?

The signs of drowning (see below) and occasionally objects such as gravel, rope or aquatic plants grasped in the hands (Fig. 6-1) are the only post mortem findings which would permit the conclusion that immersion took place during life.

The causes of death in the water

As will be shown, the diagnosis of drowing is both difficult to make and to exclude. The examiner must bear in mind other causes of death in the water which include:

(1) natural causes, particularly heart and brain lesions,

(2) asphyxia due to aspiration of stomach contents,

(3) injuries sustained while swimming (ship's propeller), diving (fractures, decompression sickness, air embolism) or falling into the water (fractures),

(4) electrocution (lightning in open bodies of water, radios or sun lamps in bathrooms, underwater lights in swimming pools) (because of the low electrical resistance of moist skin no electrical burns may be present),

(5) cardiac arrest due to sudden immersion in cold water ("immersion syndrome") (there are no diagnostic autopsy findings),

(6) injuries caused by aquatic animals, such as fish or coelenterates. These are rare and peculiar to certain geographic regions.

All of the above, when not lethal in themselves, may incapacitate the victim to such an extent that drowning follows. Severe intoxication or unconsciousness from any cause (fainting, epileptic seizure) may lead to drowning, sometimes in very shallow water. The role of respiratory alkalosis caused by voluntary over-breathing prior to diving[38]* and the hazards of scuba diving,[131, 162] such as carbon dioxide narcosis and air embolism, in contributing to accidental drownings are now being recognized.

DROWNING

In spite of the frequency of accidental drowning the nature of the lethal process is still incompletely understood and its post mortem recognition, even in fresh cases, difficult. In Canada in a typical year (1974) 1,035 accidental drownings were recorded which constituted 0.6 per cent of all deaths and 8.0 per cent of all accidental deaths. Of these 242 (23.4 per cent) were children under 15 and 289 (27.9 per cent) youths in the 15 to 24 year age group. Males outnumbered females 7 to 1.[1]

The mechanism of drowning

The old concept, held throughout the classical and medieval periods, that death in drowning was caused by the swallowing of large amounts of fluid is still reflected in the German "ertrinken". When it was recognized that fluid penetrated into the respiratory system, a purely mechanical concept was formulated according to which fluid replaced the air in the lungs resulting in a fatal lack of oxygen. It is now known that, while anoxia does play an important role, the complex biochemical and hemodynamic changes caused by the presence of water in the lung are equally important and may lead to death by mechanisms other than simple lack of oxygen.

During drowning in water, the fluid which reaches the respiratory system ranges from massive amounts to hardly detectable quantities. The latter produce the paradoxical phenomenon of "dry drowning" in which the respiratory passages appear to be free from water and the lungs dry and often distended with air (ballooning) . A reasonable, if not entirely satisfactory, explanation of this condition is that of spasm of the larynx which prevents the entrance of water and persists until after the stage of respiratory efforts.

The water which reaches the lungs is immediately exposed to a vast network of capillary blood vessels and to osmotic and ionic interchange with the circulating fluid (plasma) , the direction of such

*References are to Bibliography beginning on page 159.

interchange depending on the tonicity of the water. As long as the blood is moving through the blood vessels this is a continuous process and even in a few seconds large amounts of water can enter or leave the circulation.

In fresh water, thinning of the blood (hemodilution), increased blood volume (hypervolemia) and a breakdown of red blood cells (hemolysis) occur, the latter resulting in a sharp increase in blood potassium (hyperkalemia), while the aspiration of sea water rapidly leads to an escape of fluid from the circulation into the lungs (pulmonary edema), concentration of the blood (hemoconcentration) and a diminished blood volume (hypovolemia).

Heavily chlorinated or contaminated water may be very irritating to the lung and may evoke an acute and often fatal pneumonia several hours or even days after rescue and apparent recovery ("secondary drowning").

The various pathways which may be involved in drowning are shown in the diagram below.

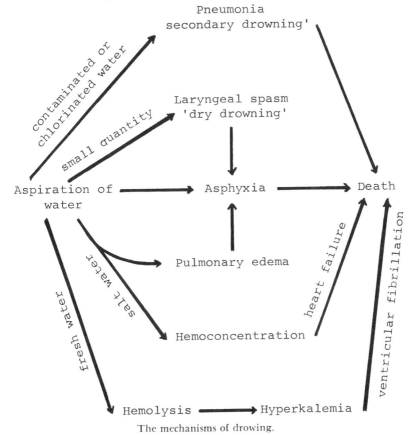

The mechanisms of drowning.

The recognition of drowning

Drowning is difficult to recognize even in those recently dead. Post mortem changes rapidly obscure even the few findings upon which the pathologist could base an opinion so that in the stage of putrefaction the diagnosis of drowning is usually one of exclusion. Below are given the findings frequently encountered in those drowned, although only a few of them may be present in a given case.

Findings indicative of drowning:

  (1) Large amounts of water in the lungs. It may occasionally be possible to characterize the water by its content of chlorine in swimming pool drownings, soap in bathwater drownings or microscopic organisms from natural bodies of water.

  (2) Diatoms in organs other than the lungs. This may be the only finding in decomposing bodies (see below).

Findings suggestive of drowning:

  (1) foam in mouth, nose and respiratory passages,

  (2) distension of the lungs with air (ballooning),

  (3) diatoms or algae in the lungs (see below),

  (4) water in the stomach,

  (5) gravel or mud in the respiratory passages, esophagus or stomach,

  (6) watery fluid in the chest cavities,

  (7) hemorrhages into the middle ears or ethmoid sinuses,

  (8) the grasping of objects in the hands (Fig. 6-1).

Findings of no value in the recognition of drowning:

  (1) absence of water in the lungs,

  (2) goose flesh,

  (3) absence of diatoms in the organs,

  (4) wrinkling of the skin of the hands and feet,

  (5) the distribution of lividity or its colour,

  (6) the presence or absence of maggots,

  (7) the floating or sinking of the body,

  (8) the chemical changes in the blood (see below).

The presence of "plankton"

When water containing particulate matter including microscopic algae or diatoms ("plankton") is aspirated, these organisms appear in the smaller air passages or even in the air sacs of the lungs (alveoli). Organisms which are very small, less than 30 microns in width, are able to enter ruptured capillary blood vessels and are carried to other organs during the last moments of life.[127, 128, 178] The main objections to their significance in the diagnosis of drowning has been the possibility that, in the case of submerged bodies, water might have entered the lungs after death and that diatoms, which have been found in dust, air and rain water, might have contaminated the organs during the autopsy.[165]

The consensus at the moment appears to be that, provided adequate precautions were taken during the dissection to prevent contamination from the air or the clothing, the findings of diatoms in the systemic circulation and in organs such as liver, brain, heart and bone marrow is evidence of drowning, that the finding of large numbers

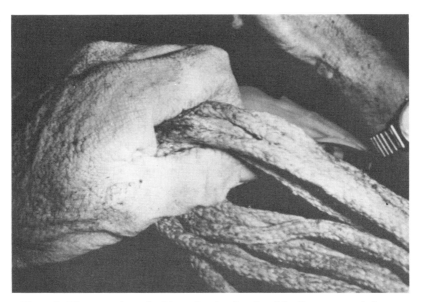

Fig. 6-1. The grasping of objects in the hands of bodies recovered from water strongly suggests that death occured in the water but gives no information concerning the cause of death.

only in the lungs indicates terminal aspiration of water irrespective of the cause of death and that the presence of a few organisms only in the lungs may represent post mortem penetration. The gaping of body cavities and the consequent exposure of the organs to the water, of course, completely invalidates these findings.

The original expectation that the types of organisms found might provide a clue to the locality of the drowning has not often borne fruit in practice as too many variables are involved. The plankton content of natural bodies of water fluctuates greatly, not only from season to season, but also during a given day. The failure to find microscopic organisms, therefore, does not exclude drowning. Furthermore, organisms are usually absent from pool and bath water.

Methods of demonstrating these organisms include the direct microscopic examination of fluid expressed from the lungs and various techniques which involve the digestion of tissue by strong acids. The latter destroy all organisms except the silicateous skeletons of the diatoms.

Blood tests in the diagnosis of drowning

The penetration of fresh water into the circulation of the lungs and the blood concentration caused by salt water, which have both been shown to occur under experimental conditions, have provided the theoretical basis for a number of chemical and physical blood tests. These include the determination of the freezing point of blood serum, blood cell volume (hematocrit), the refractive index and osmotic pressure of blood serum and the levels of chlorides and magnesium. These tests usually comprise the comparison of blood samples taken from the right and left sides of the heart.

The levels of blood chlorides (Gettler-Yamakami test) have been used most widely.[51,174] It seems, however, that a large amount of water has to be aspirated, that even a short survival time permits mixing of blood from the systemic and lung circulations and, finally, that the rapid post mortem diffusion of these substances quickly abolishes any difference in chloride levels. These tests, therefore, have been disappointing and cannot, at this time, be regarded as being of practical usefulness.[164]

How long has the body been dead? The effects of prolonged immersion

An estimate of the period of immersion in natural bodies of water, like rivers and lakes, is always difficult. The temperature to which a body is exposed largely governs the rapidity of post mortem changes and this may vary not only from one locality to another but differ at various depths of submersion. Floating bodies may be carried long distances and sink or come to the surface at irregular intervals. Furthermore, bodies which have been recovered from water tend to undergo rapid decomposition so that the time between landing the body and the examination becomes important. In the case of bodies which have been washed ashore and exposed to the air for an unknown period, only the roughest estimate is usually possible.

The post mortem changes which affect bodies in water are similar to those seen on land but proceed more slowly and in temperatures below 8°C practically cease.

The early effects of water are seen in the skin of the hands and feet which becomes grey and wrinkled ("washerwoman's hands"). This involves the fingers and toes in a few hours, the palms and soles after about one day and the entire hand or foot in about 1 to 3 days. This is followed by the gradual loss of the outer layer of the skin (epidermis) including the hair and nails over the next 7 to 14 days. As long as the epidemis of the fingertips remains the taking of fingerprints is feasible. These changes occur more slowly in regions in which the skin is protected by clothing. Even when most of the epidermis has been lost, parts may remain underneath tight collars or belts. Late changes include the formation of adipocere (see Table 1-6).

All of the above changes are not peculiar to bodies in water but may occur in any cool and moist environment.

Post mortem artefacts

Floating or submerged cadavers are subject to a large variety of post mortem artefacts, the importance of which lies in their distinction from pre mortem injuries. In rough water abrasions are common and may contain embedded gravel or sand. Lacerations and fractures may be caused by rocks, pilings and ships' propellers, the latter occasionally amputating limbs. Crushing of the skull and the rib cage may be caused by ice floes and destruction of soft tissues by fish, rodents or crustaceans. Sometimes the general nature of the injury and, in fresh bodies, the amount of associated bleeding and its microscopic appearance may suggest a pre or post mortem origin, but often such a distinction cannot be made.

The swelling of the neck during early putrefaction may cause a tight collar or tie to produce a deep circular indentation resembling a strangulation mark. Operations involved in landing the body may leave marks on it, including impressions of rope, and vigorous attempts at artificial respiration may break ribs.

Death in the bathtub

The old style of bathtub which had four vertical sides permitted the head of an unconscious or incapacitated individual to slide beneath the water. In the modern bathtub in which one end is sloping, an adult would be maintained in a semi reclining position with the head above the water level. Accidental drownings in bathtubs are thus practically confined to those who fell into the water and to children. Homicidal bathtub drownings are rare, the famous case of George Joseph Smith ("The Brides in the Bath") notwithstanding, except in the case of infants.

Most of those found dead in the bathtub have succumbed to natural causes or to accidents like carbon monoxide poisoning or electrocution by sunlamps or radios.

Was the drowning accidental?

An opinion whether a drowning was accidental, suicidal or homicidal must take into consideration all the circumstances surrounding the case, of which the medical findings are only a part. Predisposing illness, intoxication or wounds may assume great significance. It must be remembered that the tying of hands and feet with rope or wire, and even the attachment of weights, while certainly raising the suspicion of foul play, may occasionally be seen in suicides.

7

THE VICTIMS OF FIRE

In view of the great destruction which may be caused by heat it is not surprising that the examination of bodies recovered after a fire may pose formidable difficulties. As fires are occasionally set in order to destroy evidence, every body and all specimens suspected as being of human origin must be most carefully examined.

Apart from the ascertainment of the identity of the victim, questions which confront the pathologist include: Did the death occur during the fire? Was death caused by the fire? Did the victim make any attempts to escape? If not, why not? And, in the case of fragmentary remains, how many individuals are represented?

Questions concerning the origin of the fire, whether accidental or incendiary, rarely fall within the medical examination although the finding of disability or intoxication in the victim may be of obvious importance in that connection.

The state of preservation of bodies ranges from slight smoke blackening of the skin to complete ashing, most showing intermediate degrees of destruction. The difficulties in the interpretation of autopsy findings arise from the fact that heat tends to destroy evidence of pre mortem trauma while, at the same time, mimicking such injuries. It is necessary, therefore, to be familiar with the artefacts which may be brought about by intense heat and which are likely to cause difficulty.

(1) The marked dehydration and loss of tissue causes the dimensions of the body to shrink and the body weight to fall. This shrinkage may affect individual bones so that the tables relating bone measurements to stature no longer apply.

(2) The loss of skin causes loss of features, scars and tattoos as well as of skin lacerations, cuts and bruises.

(3) The skin and subcutaneous tissue may split, simulating cuts.

(4) Hair is lost quickly. Certain types of dental filling (e.g. amalgam) melt readily, while intense heat destroys the teeth.

(5) Heat causes fractures of bones including the hyoid. Fractures of the skull are particularly common and difficult to evaluate.

The vault of the skull fragments, the fragments falling out-
wards, and there is often separation of the skull sutures.
Fractures of the base of the skull or depressed fractures
arouse suspicion.

(6) Destruction of ligaments dislocates joints. This often progresses to detachment of feet, forearms, hands and fingers.

(7) Extradural collections of blood clot (brandhematom) may
occur. Its distinction from pre mortem hematoma, while
clearly important, is not always easy. The clot of the heat
artefact tends to show a high carbon monoxide content, while
that of an extradural hemorrhage sustained prior to the fire
would show a low level or absence of carbon monoxide. Still,
a pre mortem hematoma which became exposed during the
fire may absorb sufficient carbon monoxide to cause difficulty
in interpretation.

Did death occur in the fire?

Signs of efforts to escape show not only that death occurred in the
fire but that the victim was conscious at the time.

The finding of soot in the air passages is indicative of smoke inhalation. More difficult to assess is the presence of small amounts of
carbon in the lungs, particularly in smokers or persons working in a
dusty or smoky environment. The absence of carbon particles is not
informative. Particles in the nostrils or nasal passages are disregarded.

The searing of the mouth, nose or air passages by hot air, while
not always present, is a more reliable indication that breathing had
taken place during the fire.

In persons found dead after a fire the distinction between pre and
post mortem burns is usually not possible because there would generally not have been sufficient time for vital reactions to have occurred.

The finding of a significant carbon monoxide saturation of the
blood is excellent evidence that the deceased had been alive for some
time during the fire, although not necessarily conscious (see below).

Did the fire cause death?

Victims of a conflagration may succumb to a variety of insults
such as:

During the fire	Burns
	Carbon monoxide poisoning
	Accidents (falling down the stairs, being hit by débris)
	Blast injuries
	A combination of the above

Within 24 hours after rescue	Shock
	Edema of the larynx or lungs due to inhalation of hot air
	Smoke inhalation
During subsequent days or weeks	Infection
	Electrolyte imbalance
	Kidney failure
	Delayed effects of carbon monoxide poisoning
	Ulcers of the stomach or duodenum

"Spontaneous combustion", "preternatural combustibility"

The term "spontaneous combustion" refers to the spontaneous ignition and burning of a living individual or dead body without an external source of heat. While there are several reports of such an event in the older literature, none could be considered acceptable by modern criteria.

On the other hand, a number of instances have been reported in recent years in which an extensively burned body was found in largely undamaged surroundings. These usually involved elderly women, often alcoholic, and occurred near a stove or open fire place.[54,180]* It is difficult to avoid the conclusion that some factor rendered these bodies unusually ("preternaturally") combustible. Obesity, draughts and the type of clothing worn have all been incriminated.

Carbon monoxide in the blood

Carbon monoxide, which is evolved during the combustion of organic materials, is inhaled by victims of fire. While many die solely as the result of this inhalation, others are merely incapacitated, but often to such an extent that efforts to escape become ineffectual. In any event, the presence of carbon monoxide in the blood is regarded as evidence that the deceased had been alive for some time during the fire and the level of carbon monoxide attained is regarded as a rough indication of the length of that time.

The following questions concerning carbon monoxide tend to recur in court:

(1) Does the absence of carbon monoxide in the blood show that the individual died before the fire? Total absence of carbon monoxide would certainly raise the suspicion that the person had been dead at the time. However, in very rapid deaths caused by explosions or accidents at the beginning of the fire no carbon monoxide may be demonstrable.[83]

---

*References are to Bibliography beginning on page 159.

(2) Does carbon monoxide penetrate into the blood after death? The intact body surface is a very effective barrier to the penetration of carbon monoxide. During prolonged exposures to a high concentration sufficient carbon monoxide may penetrate into the capillary blood vessels of the skin to produce the typical bright red colour, but the blood in the deeper vessels will not contain carbon monoxide.[167] When the chest or abdominal cavities are open, on the other hand, considerable post mortem penetration can occur.

(3) Does the burning of the body itself produce carbon monoxide? While the burning of the body and the clothing liberates carbon monoxide into the air, blood levels are not affected.[41, 187]

(4) Does exposure to heat destroy the chemical evidence of carbon monoxide inhalation? As long as the blood remains fluid carbon monoxide determinations can be performed without difficulty. Intense heat may convert the blood into a solid, brick red substance (carboxyhemochromogen) which can also be analyzed for carbon monoxide by special techniques.

For a further discussion of carbon monoxide, see Chapter 5.

Smoke inhalation

The only significance which had, until recently, been attached to the finding of soot deposits in the air passages and lungs had been that of a vital phenomenon indicative of respiration during a fire. The expression "overcome by smoke" has been used to refer to lack of oxygen or to carbon monoxide poisoning but now the noxious nature of smoke itself is being recognised.

Hot smoke consists largely of a suspension of carbon particles, water vapour and various amounts of carbon dioxide and carbon monoxide, but may also contain lung irritants such as ammonia, aldehydes, chlorine, oxides of nitrogen and phosgene. Carbon itself is chemically inert but, as smoke cools, these irritating substances condense on the carbon particles making them intensely irritating to the lungs and the lining of the air passages. Survivors of fires may thus, several hours after rescue, develop acute, and sometimes fatal, edema of the lungs and pneumonia. Toxic gases such as hydrogen sulfide, hydrogen cyanide and methane may also be evolved, especially by the combustion of plastics and synthetic fibers.

In addition, the heat of fires may cause leakage and vaporization of stored chemicals, particularly in industrial premises, and poisoning by their inhalation.

The pathological examination of victim of fire

The methods of examination naturally depend on the degree of destruction of the body. In charred bodies the examination of the teeth frequently offers the only chance of an identification, although intense heat may burn teeth and destroy dental work. All dentures and denture fragments should be retained. Dental x-rays should be taken or, if some delay in the identification is expected, the entire dentition should be retained. The pathologist will usually have to call on the help of a forensic odontologist.

As long as the skin remains, even in a heat coagulated condition, fingerprinting may be possible (Fig. 7-1). On the other hand, heat quickly destroys the proteins of the blood, so that tests for blood groups or even the determination of the species are rarely possible in severely burned remains.

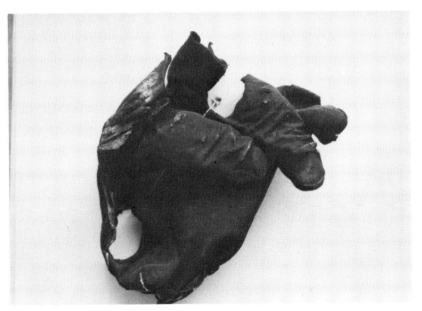

Fig. 7-1. Skin cast of the hand of a charred body from which three fingerprints could be obtained.

Burned bodies should be x-rayed and all metal objects which resemble bullets or which cannot be identified collected. Soft bullets and shot gun pellets melt at about 340°C (662°F). (The heat in house fires may reach 1500°C or 2732°F.) In the case of jacketed ammunition the hard jacket tends to remain intact but the soft core may melt.

The extent, distribution and severity of skin burns should be recorded, the severity being graded as "first degree" (reddening only), "second degree" (blistering) or "third degree" (entire skin thickness burned). An estimate of the proportion of skin surface burned should also be made.

Blood and tissue samples must be taken for carbon monoxide and alcohol determination and for the detection of drugs and poisons.

Sections for microscopic examination should be prepared from all organs and, in severely burned bodies, these must include the sex organs. Special care must be taken in cutting the lungs to avoid accidental transfer of carbon particles.

Jewellery, personal effects and clothing must be collected for expert study. If the clothing is to be tested for traces of volatile substances such as gasoline, it must be put into tightly sealed glass containers, not into plastic bags. The clothing must be searched for cuts, bullet holes or blood stains.

8

INFANTS AND CHILDREN

Depending on the circumstances, the objectives of an examination of an infant may include the determination of the cause of death, the establishment of its degree of maturity, the assessment of viability, the detection of signs of live birth and, on occasion, the tracing of its origin.

In the uterus, unless infection has been introduced by unsterile instruments, penetrating injuries or rupture of the membranes, the fetus is sterile and after its death decomposition is slow and purely autolytic in nature. It becomes evident about 24 hours after fetal death by a patchy detachment of the skin. The changes seen in the newborn infant are similar except that putrefaction may occur in tissues which had become contaminated by bacteria after birth, such as the respiratory and intestinal tracts.

Naturally, the difficulties of the examination increase as the time since death lengthens. In addition, the bodies of infants rapidly dehydrate in a dry environment and are subject to the usual destruction by insects and animals.

The cause of death

An infant's failure to survive can often be explained by immaturity or a major developmental defect such as the absence of the brain (anencephaly). The finding of lethal injuries usually presents no problem, provided the autopsy technique is adequate, particularly as far as the examination of the head is concerned. The difficulty generally lies in deciding whether the injuries found are likely to have been sustained accidentally or inflicted intentionally. It must be remembered that the process of birth itself, especially when occurring in the absence of medical assistance or under conditions of concealment, may be a very traumatic event for the infant.

Birth injuries include fractures of the skull, fractures and dislocations of long bones, rupture of the liver and tears of the venous sinuses of the dura resulting in subdural hemorrhage.[70]* The infant may be accidentally strangled by the umbilical cord or fatal hemorrhage may occur from the end of the umbilical cord. Precipitate delivery into a toilet may result in drowning. The possibility that injuries may have been inflicted during frantic but unskilled attempts at resuscitation must be kept in mind.

While it is generally true that the greater the extent and severity of the injuries, the less likely they are to have been sustained accidentally, the marks of intentional violence may be minimal. A few fingermarks or fingernail scratches on the neck may be the only finding in strangulation and some methods of child killing such as smothering, drowning in clear water or exposure, may leave no diagnostic findings at all.

The maturity of the fetus and viability

An estimate of fetal maturity may become important in cases of disputed paternity and in tracing the origin of an abandoned infant and in this the pathologist will base his opinion on several observations. Unfortunately, those most easily made, namely the body weight, body length and the circumference of the head, are also those most rapidly altered by post mortem processes. The length of the umbilical cord and the weight of the afterbirth (placenta) are too variable to provide more than a very rough guide.

The order of appearance of small islands of bone (centres of ossification) in the fetal skeleton, beginning in the collar bone (clavicle) and gradually involving other bones, is quite consistent. These centres of ossification can be demonstrated by various methods including x-ray, in the later stages, and provide a good index of fetal age even when post mortem changes are moderately advanced.

The term "viability" denotes the stage of maturity at which a normally developed infant is potentially able to survive. The term is generally used in its legal rather than in its biological sense, the legal definitions of viability ranging from 20 to 28 weeks of intra-uterine life.

Viability is, of course, not synonymous with live birth. A fetus which has reached maturity may not be viable because of a major developmental defect or a normally developed, viable infant may be stillborn because of obstetrical complications. Furthermore, very immature, "pre-viable" infants may show signs of life following birth and thus acquire a legal personality.

---

*References are to Bibliography beginning on page 159.

Live birth

Any charge of murder or of infanticide depends on proof that the infant had been alive after birth and this is often the most crucial and difficult objective of the examination. In the legal sense an infant is regarded as having been born alive if, after being completely external to the mother, it had shown any sign of life, whether or not the umbilical cord had been cut or the placenta delivered.

Of the early manifestations of life, namely heart beat, body movements and breathing or crying, only the last, which involves penetration of air into the lungs and distension of the air sacs, will leave changes which could be recognized after death.

Aeration of the lungs causes an increase of blood flow and thus an increase in the weight of the lungs. This was at one time regarded as a useful index (static test). It is now clear that there is too great an overlap of values to make this test reliable.

The lowering of the specific gravity of lung tissue due to the entry of air forms the basis of the "flotation" or "hydrostatic" test which still has limited validity. After the main air passages have been tied the lungs are removed from the body and placed on water. They will float if approximately half the lung substance has been aerated. Lesser degrees of aeration may be detected by cutting each lung into 8 to 10 pieces and observing how many of these float. Air introduced into the lung by artificial respiration and the presence of putrefactive gases, of course, invalidate this test.

The degree of aeration of the lungs during the first few hours of life is so small that even microscopic examination of the lungs may not detect it. The distinction between spontaneously inspired air and that artificially introduced may not be possible. The presence of putrefactive gases is not difficult to recognize, although at that stage it is usually impossible to be certain whether some respiratory expansion of the lungs had been present before putrefaction. It must also be remembered that infants have been known to breathe or even cry before being completely external to the mother.

Air which is swallowed during crying can be demonstrated in the stomach 5 to 15 minutes after birth, in the small intestine after 1 to 2 hours and in the large intestine after 5 to 6 hours.[85] This finding, too, is invalidated by resuscitation and putrefaction.

There are very few other findings which might help in the recognition of live birth. After its severance the umbilical cord is without blood circulation and dries and, after a few days, separates from the umbilicus. This drying, however, is a purely physical process and will occur in the dead as well as in the living infant. A moist environment, moreover, would prevent drying. In the live infant, a healing process takes place at the junction of the dead cord tissue and the underlying umbilical stump. Recognition of this vital process supplies proof of live birth but even microscopic evidence of healing does not become visible for several days.

Meconium, which is the stool in the large intestine of the newborn, is usually expelled soon after birth by the living infant, but this is not invariable and it may occur while the infant is still in the uterus or in the birth passages.

Finding that the infant had taken nourishment is, of course, proof of live birth. Jaundice and pneumonia, while usually post-natal in onset, can occur in utero and are therefore not reliable indicators of live birth.

Findings indicative of stillbirth:

    (1) maceration

Findings suggestive of stillbirth:

    (1) major developmental anomalies
    (2) marked immaturity (weight below 300 grams)

Findings suggestive of live birth:

    (1) age of viability
    (2) air in the lungs (in the absence of resuscitation or putrefaction)
    (3) air in stomach and intestine (in the absence of resuscitation)
    (4) drying of umbilical cord
    (5) absence of meconium in the intestine
    (6) pneumonia
    (7) jaundice

Findings indicative of live birth:

    (1) food in the stomach
    (2) healing of the umbilical stump

Findings of no value in distinguishing stillbirth from live birth:

    (1) rigor mortis
    (2) petechial hemorrhages
    (3) putrefaction
    (4) mummification
    (5) attached placenta
    (6) evidence of attempted child killing (e.g. ligature around the neck) .

Tracing the origin

Tracing the origin of an abandoned infant does not fall within the scope of the medical examination, although the material in which the body may have been wrapped may become important. The contribution of the pathologist consists of the determination of the cause of death, the infant's maturity and racial origin and of an estimate of the time elapsed between birth and death and between death and discovery. Specimens of blood and muscle should always be taken for the determination of blood groups.

Crib deaths

The so called "crib death", "cot death" or "sudden infant death syndrome" (S.I.D.S.) remains one of the great engimas in forensic medicine. While no definition of this condition is universally accepted, the above terms are applied to the unexpected death of an infant who appeared to have been in good health. The autopsy is either entirely negative or the findings are minimal, consisting merely of pin point hemorrhages in the thymus, over the pleura and pericardium and, occasionally, of slight edema of the lungs. In the present state of our knowledge the diagnosis of crib death is thus one of exclusion.

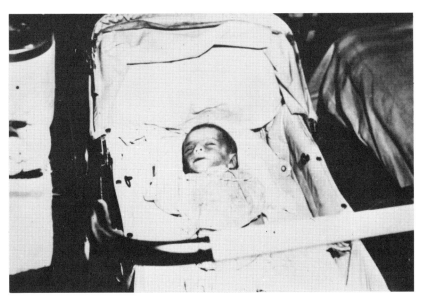

Fig. 8-1. A case regarded at first as one of crib death. The pallor of the forehead, nose and chin suggested that the child's face had been pressed against the pillow and this was eventually admitted by the mother.

This syndrome constitutes the most common type of infant death after the immediate neonatal period, the reported incidence ranging from 1 to 2 per 1000 live births. It is rare before the age of one month and after 6 months, showing a peak incidence at 3 months. Its cause remains unknown although the presence of petechial hemorrhages suggests an asphyxial mode of death. The demise of these infants tends to occur during sleep, usually at night, and appears to be not only sudden, but also gentle, as there are no signs of struggle or distress.

As might be expected, many causes have been incriminated some of which, such as enlargement of the thymus ("status thymico-lymphaticus"), suffocation by soft pillows, "overlaying" and climatic fluctuations, are now of mere historical interest. Other possibilities which are still under active study include respiratory infections, both bacterial and viral,[8, 60, 89, 173] spasm of the bronchial tubes,[171] obstruction of the nose,[171] allergy to cow's milk, anomalies of the parathyroid glands[55] and disorders of the conducting system of the heart.[87]

The immediate problem confronting the pathologist who is examining an infant who died unexpectedly is to detect both natural and accidental causes of death and, more difficult, to exclude the possibility of foul play.

The exclusion of homicide depends on meticulous autopsy technique and the careful recording of even seemingly trivial findings, such as petechial hemorrhages in the scalp, scratch marks or an unusual distribution of lividity (Fig. 8-1). It is also essential to exclude drug overdose in every case of apparent crib death by an adequate toxicological analysis.

The "battered child"

In 1946 Caffey[23] described an association of subdural hematoma and fractures in children and in 1955 Wooley and Evans[189] suggested the role of intentional maltreatment. Since then there has been a growing awareness both amongst the medical profession and the lay public of the frequency of such maltreatment, resulting in the concept of the "battered child". A gratifying result of this awareness has been the increasing recognition of these children in hospitals and doctors' offices and their gradual disappearance from the autopsy services.

There are only a few injuries which, in themselves, are indicative of maltreatment. Generally, the battered child, which is often well nourished and which may appear well cared for, will have a variety of injuries (Fig. 8-2) sustained at different times.

The information given to the hospital, police or coroner by the parents or those who had been looking after the child is notoriously unreliable and usually attributes the injuries to the child's tendency to fall or to a variety of accidents. Of course, the punctate burns caused by cigarette ends or the typical elliptical marks left by beating with a loop of rope or electric cord would be difficult to explain on that basis. Usually, however, the pathologist can merely raise the suspicion of maltreatment.

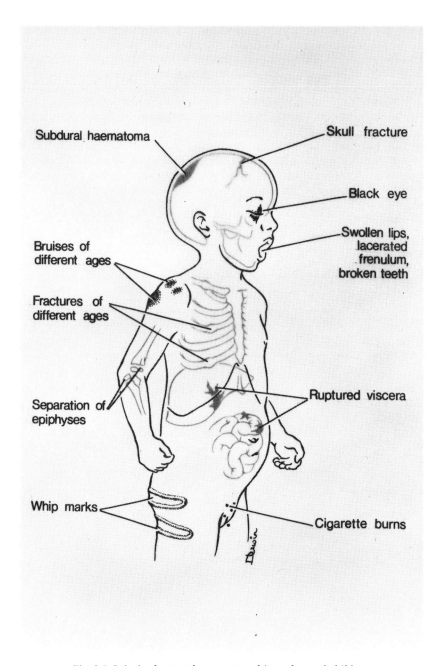

Fig. 8-2. Injuries frequently encountered in maltreated children.

While the maltreated child must be recognized, it must be remembered that children do fall and injure themselves, that they fight and get hurt and that unintended injury may result from corporal punishment administered by well meaning parents or by unskilled attempts at resuscitation. Abnormalities of the skeletal system which result in excessive brittleness of bone must be excluded because, although they are rare, this possibility may well be raised in court. The same applies to scurvy and other blood disturbances which could result in excessive bruising and to neurological disorders which would predispose to falls.

In the examination of a child that allegedly died as the result of intentional violence the nature of the injuries and the cause of death are usually quite evident. The difficulty generally lies in deciding the manner in which the injuries may have been sustained, their relative ages and in excluding any disease which could have made the child susceptible to minor degrees of violence which would have been innocuous to a normal child.

The autopsy procedure must, therefore, be meticulous and so well documented that the pathological findings could subsequently be assessed by other pathologists, including neuropathologists, as well as by specialists in other fields such as pediatrics and radiology.

The body should be weighed and measured and the entire skeleton x-rayed. All external injuries must be measured, described in detail and photographed. Colour photography may be essential in order to show differences in age between various bruises. Photographs should include views of the entire body showing the distribution of injuries and close-up views showing their details.

All internal injuries must be described in detail and photographed. It is advisable to keep the organ or organs upon which the diagnosis of the cause of death has been based until the conclusion of all legal proceedings.

Tissue blocks for microscopic study, carefully labelled, should be taken from all external injuries, fracture sites and internal injuries, as well as from uninjured parts of the skeleton, from bone marrow, spleen and spinal cord. Adequate specimens for toxicological analysis should also be collected.

For an excellent review of the medical as well as the social aspects of the problem of maltreated children see Cameron, Johnson and Camps.[24]

Poisoning in children

Poisoning in infancy is not common. The few cases which are seen are usually due to the inadvertent addition of toxic substances, such as boric acid, to the food or the accidental substitution of salt for sugar. The administration of excessive amounts of sedative to the infant by the parents or the baby sitter accounts for a few additional cases.

In older children, on the other hand, especially in the age period from 1 to 4 years, accidental poisoning is so common that it must always be suspected in a sudden death of an apparently well child. It is during this stage of development that the child acquires mobility and manual dexterity and passes through a period of great inquisitiveness.

The toxic substances involved are thus those commonly found in the house, particularly in medicine cabinets, in the garage and in the garden. To the latter must be added poisonous berries and mushrooms.

In a typical year in Canada,[22] 32,265 poisonings were reported in children below the age of 5, representing 68.3 per cent of all poisonings. Acetylsalicylic acid ("aspirin") and its preparations were by far the most common source, constituting 24 per cent of poisonings in these children. This was followed by cleaning and polishing agents (14 per cent), central nervous system drugs such as tranquillizers, sedatives and narcotics (7 per cent), cosmetics (7 per cent), respiratory drugs (5 per cent), paints and building products (4.5 per cent) and gastro-intestinal drugs (4 per cent). The death rate was 2.3 per cent, a sharp decline from recent years probably reflecting the increasing availability and effectiveness of poison control centres.

9

ASPHYXIA.
COMPRESSION OF THE NECK

Many conditions of forensic interest have as their final lethal pathway a lack of oxygen, either because of an inadequate oxygen supply or because of an inability of the tissues to use oxygen. The collective term "asphyxia" is generally applied to these conditions and, while the term literally means "pulselessness", it seems too firmly established to be replaced by the more accurate terms "anoxia" or "hypoxia". It must be clearly understood that "asphyxia" signifies a terminal state of oxygen lack and not the manner in which such a state was brought about. "Asphyxia" without qualification is not an acceptable pathological diagnosis.

The deprivation of oxygen may occur at the following levels:

(1) the breathing of an atmosphere devoid of oxygen or containing oxygen at a partial pressure of less than 40 millimetres of mercury (industrial accidents, scuba diving accidents, failure of oxygen supply in, or depressurization of, an aircraft, mountain sickness, mishaps during surgical anaesthesia),

(2) prevention of respiratory movements (traumatic asphyxia, crushing injuries of the chest, poisoning by organophosphates),

(3) obstruction of airway (smothering, choking, strangulation),

(4) impairment of oxygen diffusion in the lung (drowning, edema of the lungs),

(5) impairment of oxygen transport (obstruction of blood circulation, shock, carbon monoxide poisoning),

(6) interference with oxygen use by the tissues (low blood sugar, cyanide poisoning),

(7) injury or depression of the respiratory centre of the brain (trauma, increased intracranial pressure, drug overdose).

The clinical effects of acute lack of oxygen

Contrary to popular opinion, the simple lack of oxygen is not distressing to the victim. If it is sudden, rapid unconsciousness ensues

(Fig. 9-1), if gradual, a feeling of well being (euphoria) is followed by drowsiness, coma and death.

Great distress, on the other hand, causing the victim to make frenzied efforts to extricate himself, results when the exhalation of carbon dioxide is prevented (choking, smothering) or when there is localized pressure on the voice box or wind pipe (strangulation).

Individuals show a great range of susceptibility to lack of oxygen. Infants up to the age of about 4 months are relatively resistant and so are patients who have suffered from slowly progressive conditions resulting in chronic hypoxia, such as emphysema of the lungs. The effects depend on the degree and duration of oxygen deprivation and the body's oxygen requirements. The latter largely depends on the type of physical activity and the body temperature.

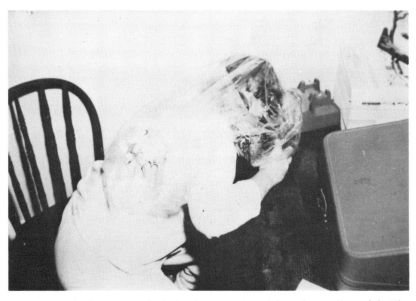

Fig. 9-1. Death due to simple lack of oxygen is quick and not distressful. The plastic bag accidentally slipped over the young woman's face while she was speaking on the telephone

The post mortem diagnosis of asphyxia

The diagnosis of asphyxia after death is always uncertain, not only because the tissue changes are non-specific, but because death often occurs too rapidly for any recognizable changes to appear. Furthermore, the recognition of terminal anoxia per se is of limited value because death from many causes is preceded by lack of oxygen.

Organs differ in their oxygen requirements. The brain is the most likely organ to sustain damage because in adults it requires 20 to 25 per cent of the oxygen breathed and in children about 50 per cent. Irreparable brain damage usually occurs in 4 to 5 minutes of complete oxygen deprivation at normal body temperature. Although some parts of the brain are more vulnerable than others, the distribution or severity of brain damage is unpredictable in a given case.

Other tissues are much less sensitive to oxygen lack. The organ next in order of susceptibility, the kidney, possesses, unlike the brain, a great capacity for regeneration and repair following anoxic damage.

The appearance of the blood. The colour of the blood reflects its oxygen content. Normally during life arterial blood with a saturation of 97 per cent is bright red; venous blood with a saturation of about 75 per cent is darker. In asphyxial states the terminal oxygen saturation may be considerably below this so that the blood is strikingly dark.

The traditional view that the presence of fluid blood indicated an asphyxial mode of death can no longer be maintained. In a cadaver the processes of clotting and liquefaction of blood occur simultaneously, sometimes one of them predominating. Most fresh cadavers will thus show a mixture of fluid and clotted blood. Mole[122]* has shown that the blood in many cases of sudden death, irrespective of cause, was fluid and not coagulable. In cases of dying slowly of infection or wasting, the clotting process predominated. Apart from indicating a sudden type of death, fluidity of the blood gives no further information.

Petechial hemorrhages. These are minute bleeding points in the skin or the mucous or serous membranes. They have long been regarded as characteristic of asphyxia, particularly those on the lungs and the pericardial sac which have acquired the eponym "Tardieu's spots".

These petechial hemorrhages are caused by local tissue anoxia and are especially common in areas in which the venous outflow is obstructed, for instance by a ligature.

Petechial hemorrhages are seen in many pathological conditions marked by terminal lack of oxygen and congestion, such as heart failure, and are, therefore, not diagnostic of any particular type of asphyxia. Their number is not important but their distribution may indicate a level of venous obstruction, such as constriction of the neck or compression of the chest.

It must also be remembered that petechial hemorrhages may appear after death. Post mortem petechial hemorrhages can, of course,

---

*References are to Bibliography beginning on page 159.

occur only in regions in which the capillary blood vessels contain blood. On the skin, therefore, they are confined to areas of lividity but internally their distribution is less predictable.

Cyanosis. This is a blue discolouration which appears on the skin and mucous membranes when the oxygen saturation of capillary blood falls below 70 per cent. It is most noticeable in the lips, tip of the nose, earlobes and fingertips. In the cadaver, some reduction of the oxygen saturation occurs supravitally during the first few hours after death so that some degree of cyanosis is seen in most cadavers. Again, many diseases, especially those of a respiratory or circulatory nature, show cyanosis in their terminal stages so that it cannot be regarded as diagnostic of asphyxia in the forensic sense.

Other post mortem findings, such as congestion of organs, dilatation of the heart chambers and edema of the lungs, are also too nonspecific to be of diagnostic value.

It is unfortunate that the three classical signs upon which the diagnosis of asphyxia had been based, namely the fluidity of the blood, petechial hemorrhages and cyanosis, are no longer valid and that no more reliable signs have been found. Efforts to find consistent chemical changes which would permit the post mortem recognition of anoxic states[12, 13, 98, 120] have not, so far, provided any practical help.

Smothering

Fatal anoxia brought about by the occlusion of the mouth and nostrils is known as "smothering" or by the older term "suffocation". Accidental smothering is seen in infants in whose cribs plastic laundry bags have been used as waterproof sheets and in the rare instances of "overlaying". In adults it is encountered in intoxicated individuals who have fallen into soft bedding or mud, and during autoerotic practices employing plastic bags. Suicidal smothering had been practically unknown until the introduction of plastic bags but nowadays it is not uncommon.

Homicidal smothering is not common and is largely confined to children and to intoxicated or incapacitated victims.

The autopsy diagnosis of smothering is usually one of considerable difficulty. The face may be congested and show evidence of having been pressed against a soft surface or object (Fig. 8-1) and the deep surface of the scalp may show petechial hemorrhages. The head and neck may show injuries caused by the assailant applying pressure from behind. The mouth or nose may contain textile fibers and the inner surfaces of the lips may be contused or lacerated by pressure against the teeth. Still, the diagnosis of smothering must often remain one of exclusion.

Any object which might have been used in smothering, such as a pillow or sheet, must be examined for cells, traces of blood or saliva. The importance of obtaining samples of blood and swabs from the mouth at autopsy is evident.

Choking

This term denotes the occlusion of the upper air passages to an extent which impairs respiration. It is usually accidental. In epileptics or deeply unconscious persons the tongue may obstruct, while massive aspiration of stomach contents is typically seen in alcoholics. Children are notoriously liable to aspirate foreign bodies such as small toys and peanuts. Impaction of a denture may follow a blow to the face and the hazards of surgery on the mouth and throat include the aspiration of teeth, surgical swabs and blood clots. Choking is not an uncommon mode of death in sensitivity reactions in which the lining of the larynx may swell, obstructing the intake of air.

Suicidal choking is rare and is seen only in mental patients, but choking by means of towels or wads of paper is a common method of killing newborn infants.

An interesting and relatively common example of accidental choking is the impaction of a bolus of inadequately chewed food in the inlet of the larynx, the so-called "café coronary", which usually occurs during a hearty meal in an inebriated individual. While in most instances of choking death is due to anoxia, in this particular event death is often so sudden that a vagal reflex is probably involved.

The autopsy diagnosis of choking is not difficult except in epileptics or when the gag has been intentionally removed. In examining the larynx care must be taken not to dislodge any impacted object but it is equally important not to be misled by post mortem spilling of gastric contents which may occur during the handling and transportation of the body.

The aspiration of gastric contents

During the process of vomiting a reflex normally closes the larynx and prevents the inhalation of the vomited material, but in the absence of this protective reflex gastric contents are very likely to enter the respiratory system. It is, therefore, not a rare event in debilitated states (drug overdose, alcoholic intoxication), during unconsciousness (head injuries, general anaesthesia) and in certain nervous disorders.

When the aspirated material is copious and firm in consistency it tends to block the airway and to lead to rapid asphyxia. Even an "empty" stomach, however, contains some strongly acid fluid which, when aspirated, is extremely irritating to lung tissue causing an acute pneumonia. This course of events is sometimes known as "Mendelson's syndrome"[39, 119] and may cause death some hours or days after the aspiration.

Compression of the neck

In view of the many vital structures located in the neck it is easy to understand that pressure on the area is likely to be hazardous, although the suddenness of death often comes as a surprise to assailant and victim.

The physical evidence of violence to the neck and its effects depend not only on the degree of force exerted but also on the means employed and on the anatomical level involved, whether the force was localized or constricting and whether it was intermittent or constant.

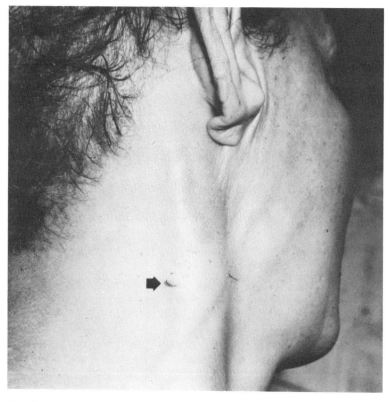

Fig. 9-2. A case of manual strangulation in which death appeared to have been due to cardiac arrest. The external marks consisted of a single fingernail scratch (arrow) and there was no internal bruising.

A constricting force of moderate severity will occlude the air passages and obstruct the veins from the head. The face will, therefore, be congested, often with petechial hemorrhages, and there may be swelling of the conjunctiva of the eyes. A severe constricting force will, in addition, obstruct the arterial blood supply to the head and, if applied quickly, the parts above the constriction will be pale without petechial hemorrhages. Rarely even slight localized force on the sides or front of the neck may kill instantly by cardiac arrest due to stimulation of the vagus nerves. In such cases there may be no, or only minimal, findings (Fig. 9-2).

The injuries to the spine of the neck and to the brain stem which are occasionally seen in "long drop" hangings and which used to be the typical findings in judicial executions, are caused by a sudden hyperextension of the neck rather than by constriction.

For a discussion of the anatomy of the neck and the effects of pressure on it see Camps and Hunt,[28] for critical reviews of the pathological findings Walcher[184] and Mosinger.[126]

For practical purposes the cases fall into two main categories, that of ligature strangulation, of which hanging is a variant, and manual strangulation. Much rarer are assaults from behind in which the neck may be compressed between the arm and forearm of the assailant and accidental falls wedging the neck between fence posts or bars of a play pen.

While the main interest focuses on the structures of the neck, injuries to other parts of the body may throw light upon the preceding events. These include bruising of the front of the body made by the knees of the attacker or signs of blows to the head.

Hemorrhages into the muscles of the neck and into the soft tissues of the spine are easily produced during the autopsy and are then indistinguishable from pre mortem injuries.[143] The importance of avoiding such artefacts is obvious.

If any injury to the spine of the neck is suspected, x-ray plates of the region should be taken before the dissection and the involved segment of the spine retained. In all instances of violence to the neck, the spinal cord, or at leasts its neck portion, must be examined.

Manual strangulation

When the neck is compressed with one hand, the thumb is placed on one side, the fingers on the other and the larynx is narrowed by side to side pressure. When both hands are used the thumbs are in front and the fingers on either side of the neck and the main force is applied from the front compressing the wind pipe and forcing the tongue backwards.

External injuries are likely to be prominent, especially if during a struggle the grip was applied repeatedly. Bruising of the skin is usually caused by the fingers of the assailant while fingernail scratches may be caused by either the assailant or the victim. Those produced by the victim are said to have a generally downward direction, those of the attacker an upward direction, but this may be difficult to ascertain in a given case. In any event, as Shapiro[157] found, the direction of application as deduced from fingernail marks may be erroneous.

Internal bruising is also likely to be severe and may consist of hemorrhage into the subcutaneous tissues and muscles of the neck, the tissues of the larynx and the spine. Post mortem changes during putrefaction make these injuries increasingly difficult to recognize.

Fractures of the hyoid bone and the thyroid cartilage have acquired the undeserved reputation of being diagnostic of manual strangulation. Fractures of these structures are found in most cases,[104] especially in the older age groups in which they are rigid, but they may not be broken, even after considerable force, in young individuals. Furthermore, fractures may occasionally be seen in other forms of strangulation and as the result of direct violence such as a karate chop. Fractures of the thyroid cartilage are actually more frequently caused by a direct blow than by compression.[28]

Death in manual strangulation is generally due to obstruction of the airway although rarely cardiac arrest may be induced by light pressure. As obstruction of the neck veins is apt to be incomplete or intermittent, and as the obstruction is relieved after death, congestion of the face and petechial hemorrhages are usually not prominent.

In the pathological examination meticulous recording of the external and internal findings is essential. The distance between the marks on the right and left sides of the neck may give a rough indication of the span of the grip. The neck organs must be removed with great gentleness in order not to produce fractures. Following their removal, the neck organs should be x-rayed before being examined further.

Ligature strangulation

The appearance of the neck in ligature strangulation depends on the nature of the ligature and the force with which it was applied. The mark tends to be more or less horizontal and may show localized depressions corresponding to knots or buckles.

Strings, ropes and belts leave uniform impressions often with a characteristic pattern which may be more evident when viewed under oblique illumination. Marks produced by towels, scarves and stockings are more irregular and less distinct.

Unless death has been very sudden, the face is congested with petechial hemorrhages. Apart from the ligature mark itself, external injuries and internal bruising are not likely to be prominent, although fingernail scratches made by the victim are not uncommon. Fractures occur rarely. The great majority of ligature strangulations are homicidal but self stranglation is not unknown.

If the ligature is still in place it should be removed without disturbing the knot. In the case of stockings and scarves this can be done by dividing it between two ties. If the ligature had been removed the strangulation mark must be described in great detail and photographed. Camps[28] recommends the use of transparent Scotch tape on the ligature mark in order to pick up any textile fibers.

Hanging

This differs from ligature strangulation only in that the ligature is attached to a fixed point and that the constricting force is due to gravity. The body need not be freely suspended but may be standing, sitting or even lying.

The ligature mark tends to be oblique rising towards the point of suspension, usually at the back of the head or behind the ears.

The lesions produced and their effects are determined by the magnitude of the constricting force and the suddenness of its application. While in the relatively uncommon "long drop" hangings the main mechanism is that of sudden hyperextension of the neck resulting in dislocation of the neck vertebrae and injury to the brain stem, the constricting force may nevertheless be so severe as to fracture the larynx and tear the carotid arteries.

In the more common course of events the constriction is sufficient to occlude the airway and the arterial blood supply to the head. A pull of a mere 3.5 kilograms (7.7 pounds) will occlude the carotid arteries and a pull of 16 kilograms (35.2 pounds) the vertebral arteries as well.[153]

The face may be congested with petechial hemorrhages or pale, depending on the suddenness of death. Desperate efforts of the victim to free himself may cause rope marks on the hands or forearms or bruises or scratches on the neck.

Hanging is nearly always suicidal in adults. Accidental suspension occurs in children during play and in adults during abnormal sexual practices.

The possibility of dealing with a homicidal or simulated hanging, although remote, haunts every investigator. In homicidal hangings, in addition to the signs of suspension, there are usually disabling injuries or incapacitating degrees of intoxication. The recognition of post mortem or simulated hanging depends on the finding of another cause of death or certain post mortem changes, such as a distribution of lividity which would be incompatible with vital suspension.

There are no laboratory tests which would aid in the distinction between pre and post mortem hanging. A higher level of histamine has been reported in the tissue of pre mortem ligature marks,[49] but this determination is technically difficult and not generally available. The microscopic study of ligature marks is not likely to be rewarding.

10

SEXUAL ASSAULTS

In the reconstruction of the activities of an individual shortly prior to death questions concerning recent sexual contact occasionally arise but they always become prominent in the investigation of assaults which may have been sexually motivated. In fatal cases the lethal injuries naturally assume primary importance but signs of recent sexual contact may throw light upon the motive and aid in the conviction or exoneration of suspects.

Many such assaults clearly reveal their sexual nature by involving actual or attempted intercourse but in others it is merely indicated by the location of the injuries (breasts, genitalia), by bite marks or by extreme violence or sadism. It is likely that other forms of aggressive behaviour, such as wife beating and the maltreatment of children, also belong to the general category of sexually motivated assaults.

The pathologist is alerted to the sexual nature of an assault by the type and location of the injuries and by the presence of semen but his findings are supplemented by observations at the scene and by the examination of clothing or bedding.

Semen

The thick, viscous, yellowish-grey secretion which forms the ejaculate is known as semen. It consists of cells, the sperm cells or spermatozoa, which are formed in the testes and the seminal fluid which is derived from the seminal vesicles and the prostate gland.

The volume of the ejaculate ranges from 0.2 to 6.6 millilitres with an average of 3.4 millilitres. It is fluid immediately after ejaculation, coagulates within two minutes and then re-liquifies in the subsequent 15 minutes.

Spermatozoa. These are the male germ cells and consist essentially of a small oval head and a long delicate tail. They are quite unlike any other body cells and can, in the intact state, be recognized microscopically without difficulty. There are about 100 million spermatozoa

Table 10-1
The Persistence of Spermatozoa

Living individual	Motile	Vagina	Up to 8 hours (average 3 hours) Slightly longer during menstruation?[149,151,159]*
		Cervix, uterus	Up to 110 hours (cervix),[141,149,156] 48 hours (uterus)[141]
		Rectum	No data
	Non-motile	Vagina	Up to 14 hours,[149,151,159] 6 days[37]
		Cervix, uterus	Up to 72 hours (cervix)[156]
		Rectum	Less than 24 hours[141]
Cadaver	Motile	Vagina	Up to 3 hours[141]
	Non-motile	Vagina	Up to 3 weeks[14, 141, 142, 159] depending on absence of putrefaction. In the *Christie* case up to 70 days[27]
		Cervix, uterus	No data
		Rectum	No data

*References are to Bibliography beginning on page 159.

per millilitre of ejaculate but even in normal individuals counts may range from 60 to 150 million. There are marked differences in sperm count not only between individuals but also between ejaculates from a given individual depending largely on the length of preceding abstinence.

The structure of spermatozoa of different mammalian species conforms to the same basic pattern but the details of each species are unique so that human sperm can be identified as such by microscopic examination alone.

In the vagina, spermatozoa are actively motile during the first few hours and while this is a common finding in the examination of living patients, autopsies are not usually performed during this brief period of motility. After several hours the spermatozoa shed their tails but their naked heads can still be recognized by a skilled observer.

The periods during which spermatozoa have been detected by various observers are summarized in Table 10-1. Many uncertainties are involved including the techniques of obtaining and examining the samples and the skill of the observers. These data must, therefore, be taken *cum grano salis* and be regarded as a rough guide only.

The finding of sperm cells in vaginal washings is presumptive evidence of penetration and emission during the offence, subject to the qualification that they may have been introduced by other means, e.g. on fingers. On the other hand, even if penetration and emission have taken place, spermatozoa may be absent because of an excessively long time since intercourse, their removal by douching or by the lack of sperm cells in the semen. The latter may be due to an inability of the male to produce sperm (azoospermia) or to the effects of vasectomy.

Seminal fluid. This fluid, which contains many organic and inorganic substances, is not affected by vasectomy. From the practical point of view its important constituents are proteins which enable its human origin to be established, some enzymes and group specific substances.

The enzyme acid phosphatase is found in many body cells but the only secretion which contains it in significant amounts is seminal fluid. The finding of acid phosphatase in more than trace amounts is strong evidence of emission even in the absence of spermatozoa. It is now known that small amounts of acid phosphatase may normally be present in vaginal fluid[116] and attempts have been made to distinguish this vaginal enzyme from the prostatic enzyme by electrophoresis.[2] Large amounts of acid phosphatase are always of seminal origin.

How long the enzyme persists in the living body is not known with certainty but Enos and co-workers[45] were unable to detect it after 12 hours and Pinto[137] after 40 hours. No controlled studies have been reported concerning its persistence in the cadaver. In the dried state it is extremely stable, Pinto[138] demonstrating it after 35 years on clothing.

Attempts have been made to relate the activity of the enzyme to the time since intercourse[137] but there are great individual differences in the amount of enzyme secreted, differences which may be, at least in part, dependent on age (Table 10-2), although in a given individual the acid phosphatase level in the seminal fluid seems fairly constant.

Table 10-2

Acid phosphatase activity of the prostate gland*

(King—Armstrong Units per Gram of Fresh Tissue)

Birth	4.5
4 years	1.5
13 years	73.0
Adults	522 – 2284

To what extent acid phosphatase activity may be introduced into a decomposing cadaver by putrefactive bacteria or by the infesting fauna, especially maggots, is a largely unexplored field, but Prokop[144] found large amounts of the enzyme in the secretion of a common European snail (Helix pomatia).

For a review of the laboratory aspects of acid phosphatase see Kind.[93]

Choline. The substance choline is not present in semen when freshly shed but is produced by enzymes from other substances soon after. It combines with iodides to form characteristic crystals and this is the basis of a simple test (Florence test). As other body fluids may also contain choline this test is not specific for semen.

Group specific substances. Individuals are assigned to one of the four major blood groups according to the antigenic make-up of the red blood cells. If the red blood cells contain the antigen A, the person is said to belong to blood group A, if the red cells contain antigen B, to blood group B, if the red cells contain both A and B, to blood group AB and if the red cells contain neither antigen, to blood group O. The H substance, which is the precursor of both A and B antigens, is present to some extent in all four blood groups, most abundantly in group O.

In about 80 per cent of the population, the so-called "secretors", these substances also appear in the body fluids. As they are slightly altered in these fluids they are generally referred to as "group specific substances". A secretor belonging to blood group A will secrete the group specific substances A and H in the seminal fluid, a group B secretor B and H, an AB secretor A, B and H and a group O secretor group specific substance H only.

---

*From Guttman and Guttman, see nr. 72 in Bibliography.

The same, of course, applies to the female who, if a secretor, will secrete group specific substances in the cervical and vaginal secretions. Therefore, in order to assess fully the serological findings in vaginal washings, it is necessary to know the blood group and secretor status of the accused and the blood group of the victim and sometimes the secretor status of the victim as well.

It is clear that the value of the serological findings in seminal fluid, just like blood group studies in cases of disputed paternity, lies in the exoneration of suspects. Thus, if only A and H group specific substances due to seminal fluid are found in vaginal washings they could not have come from a suspect belonging to blood groups, B, AB or O or from a group A non-secretor. They must have been derived from a secretor belonging to blood group A which comprises approximately 36 per cent of male Caucasians or 21 per cent of male Negroes.

Phosphoglutomutase. Recently the enzyme phosphoglutomutase has been used in attempts to trace the origin of seminal fluid. This enzyme which occurs in the red blood cells is secreted by most individuals in the seminal and vaginal fluid. There are three common types of this enzyme and the type in the seminal or vaginal fluid is always the same as that in the red blood cells. It is clear that the enzyme in vaginal washings can be recognized as being of seminal origin only if it is of a type different from that of the female.[148] Again, the value of phospho-glutomutase typing lies in the exoneration of suspects.

The hymen

This is a thick, roughly circular membrane which surrounds the vaginal opening. Its two surfaces are covered by mucous membrane supported by connective tissue rich in blood vessels.

While normal sexual intercourse in adult women usually leaves no marks, the first intercourse frequently produces tears of the hymen or of the skin of the vulva below the hymen. In sexual assaults, particularly those involving children, evidence of violence is usually found, ranging from small tears of the hymen to mutilating injuries including tears of the vagina.

The question which is often asked in court concerning the "virginity" of the victim must be answered with circumspection. There may be little difficulty when dealing with very young girls, but in the case of adults penetration may occur without lacerating the hymen and healed tears may have been caused by medical procedures. An intact hymen, therefore, is not proof of virginity nor are lacerations proof of the opposite.

The edges of a tear of the hymen heal quickly but do not unite. Gross evidence of recent injury has usually disappeared after one week and microscopic evidence after two weeks.

The pathological investigation of sexual assaults

The investigation of the scene is a police responsibility but the impression the pathologist may gain is invaluable, especially as far as the position of the body and the arrangement of the clothing are concerned.

The clothing must be removed carefully, each item being placed into a separate container. It must be recorded whether buttons were done up, undone or torn. Great care must be taken not to tear clothing during removal or to allow it to fall on the floor.

All injuries, no matter how trivial, must be described in detail, particularly any lesions suggestive of bite marks. These descriptions should be supplemented by close-up photographs which include a scale.

Any deposits on the skin suggestive of moist or dried semen are removed by scraping and collected in a clean glass container. The hands and fingers are examined for grasped objects, such as buttons, hairs and textile fibers. Fingernail scrapings are taken.

Specimens of scalp hair are taken by plucking. The pubic hair should be examined for dried semen and any matted areas removed with scissors. The pubic hair is gently combed with a fine comb and any loose hairs collected. A sample of pubic hair is then taken by plucking.

The mouth is inspected for lacerations. The teeth are examined for hairs and fibers. The mouth cavity is then gently washed with a small amount of water and the washings examined for spermatozoa. The washings may also be used to determine the secretor status of the victim, provided there is no massive contamination by blood.

Any injury to the anal region is noted and swabs are taken and examined for spermatozoa. The back is inspected for bruising. A number of parallel longitudinal cuts into the skin and subcutaneous tissues of the back may reveal deep bruising which, in the early post mortem period, may not be visible externally.

The vagina is gently washed with as small an amount of water or saline as possible in order to keep the dilution low. The washings are collected in a clean glass container without fixative. Swabs may be taken instead of washings but spermatozoa are more likely to disintegrate and swabs are less suitable for chemical and serological testing.

The external genitalia are examined before the body is opened. The hymen is inspected for recent or healed tears and the tightness of the vaginal opening is determined.

11

STABS AND CUTS

Wounds which are greater in depth than in width are said to be penetrating. They are seen in their purest form, sometimes called "punctures", when made by such objects as nails, needles, ice picks or closed scissors. When inflicted by such weapons as knives or open scissors which, in addition to a point, possess sharp edges, an element of cutting is also involved and the term "stab" or "stab wound" is usually employed. Penetrating injuries are commonly sustained in assaults, less commonly in accidents such as impalement on a fence, falls on objects carried in the hand or in the pocket or by being struck by a vehicle (car hood ornament).

This type of injury generally causes death by bleeding from lacerated blood vessels or from injury to the heart. Depending on the size and type of vessel severed, the bleeding may be brisk and rapidly lethal or slow and sometimes intermittent. Even penetrating wounds of the heart may only bleed slowly and permit survival for several days or even recovery. Of particular interest are penetrating injuries which merely incise the outer layers of the wall of a major artery. Bleeding may not occur at the time of injury, but the incised area, which constitutes a weak spot in the vessel wall, may gradually form a bulging (traumatic aneurysm) and this may rupture, often years after the original injury.

Death may also result from other internal injuries. The digestive tract may be perforated and peritonitis may follow, air entry into the chest cavities will cause the lungs to collapse, and the brain may be injured by stab wounds of the head. Even small lacerations of the head, neck and upper limbs may permit air to be sucked into the circulation, particularly if the victim is in the upright position, leading to air embolism.

The positions of the victim and assailant, the nature of the weapon, the force required to produce the penetration, the number, depth and direction of the injuries and the possibility of accidental or intentional self infliction are more often issues in court than the cause of death itself. These matters will therefore be briefly discussed below.

The examination of the clothing is an essential part of the autopsy and should be done by the pathologist while it is still in situ. The number and location of cuts in the clothing must be compared with the injuries on the body. Considerable information may thus be gained concerning the position of the limbs and attitude of the body as well as the arrangement of the clothing itself at the time of the event. Any opinion regarding the force needed to produce the injuries must, of course, take into consideration the type of material penetrated. Additional examination of the clothing for blood stains etc. may be carried out later in the laboratory.

The nature of the instrument

Stab wounds of the skin by instruments with a long, flat blade, like knives, are usually not difficult to recognize. In single edged weapons the sharp edge produces a clean cut while the blunt back of the blade tears the tissue causing the characteristic "fish tail" appearance, thus indicating the orientation of the blade. Any twisting of the weapon will obscure these features.

Round instruments leave small round puncture wounds which are easily overlooked, especially as there may be little or no external bleeding (Fig. 11-1).

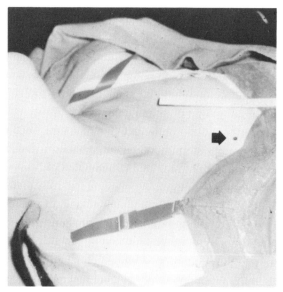

Fig 11-1. Wound of the chest by an ice pick (arrow). Note the absence of external bleeding.

Some indication of the width of the blade may be gained from the length of the surface wound, but the elasticity of the skin will tend to lead to an under-estimate while any twisting or cutting would tend to exaggerate the apparent width. In any event, it is only possible to give an estimate of the minimum width of the blade.

Only if the instrument has penetrated into a solid organ, such as the liver, will it be possible to ascertain the nature of its tip and the degree of tapering.

The number and location of wounds

The number of surface wounds must be recorded and compared with the number of cuts in the clothing. Wounds in concealed areas like the mouth, the arm pits or the anus are easily overlooked. It must also be remembered that a single thrust may produce several wounds, for example by passing through an arm into the chest, that surface wounds may be superimposed and that several thrusts may be made through a single surface wound, particularly in suicides.

The location of wounds is of importance not only in assessing the probability of accidental or intentional self infliction but also, when grouped in certain areas, in suggesting the motive of the assailant.

The depth and direction of wounds

An accurate measurement of the depth of penetration is not possible unless the wound has reached a solid structure such as the liver or the spine. Even then the fact that the abdominal and chest walls can be depressed and that organs like the heart tend to be closer to the front of the body in the erect than in the supine position must be taken into consideration. To deduce the length of the blade from the depth of penetration involves more uncertainties. Only if the skin bears an impression of the handle of the weapon, and this is rarely the case when wounds pass through clothing, is it possible to be certain that the entire blade had been inserted. It is, therefore, generally only possible to give an estimate of the minimum length of the blade.

The direction of wounds may be demonstrated by the gentle insertions of probes, avoiding the making of artificial tracks and keeping in mind the somewhat different anatomical relationships in the erect and lying positions.

The sequence of wounds

Only occasionally, when the blade has been bent or broken by striking a bone, will it be possible to determine the sequence in which the wounds were inflicted.

The difficulty of deducing the nature of the weapon from the appearance of the wounds is illustrated in Fig. 11-2. A given blade may produce a large variety of wounds depending on the degree of force employed, the twisting of the weapon and the movement of the victim's body.

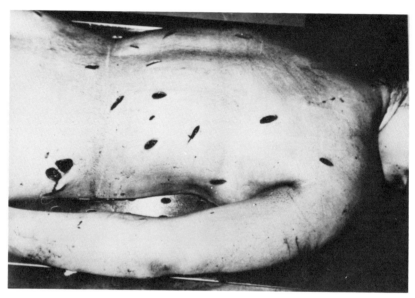

Fig. 11-2. Although these stab wounds differ greatly in appearance and depth of penetration they were all made by the same instrument.

Cuts, also known as incised wounds or slashes, are basically similar to stab wounds but differ in having a length greater than their depth. They may be made by any sharp object, but usually by metal or glass. An instrument having both a point and an edge may inflict wounds of both the stab and incised types. Undercutting of the margins of the wound occurs in oblique cuts and is a useful indicator of their direction. When made by a sharp edge the margins of a cut are "clean" but may be finely ragged when made by a blunt instrument. Serrated knives leave a characteristic appearance which may serve to identify the weapon. Because of the elasticity of the skin a cut tends to gape and external bleeding to be profuse.

Cuts are generally not difficult to identify, but must be distinguished from splits of the skin which are produced by the forceful compression of the skin against bone by a blunt object or hard surface. Unlike cuts, splits have contused margins and frequently show "bridging" of the tissue defect by tissue fibers or blood vessels. Furthermore, hairs remain intact when the skin splits, but are often cut when the skin is incised.

Are the injuries homicidal or suicidal?

The distinction between homicidal and suicidal wounds often cannot be made with certainty because, as Simpson[175a]* points out, while not all homicidal wounds can be made by a suicide, all suicidal wounds could have been inflicted by a murderer.

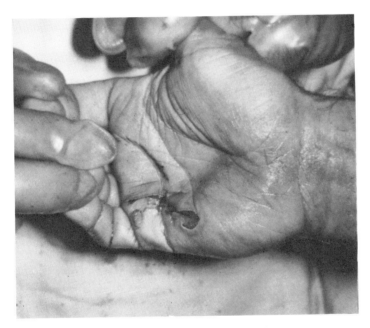

Fig. 11-3. Typical defence wounds.

Suicidal wounds must, of course, be located in a region accessible to the individual. While a multiplicity of wounds favours an assault, multiple wounds, even if several are of a lethal nature, are not incompatible with suicide. Several cuts or thrusts made through a single surface wound are strongly suggestive of self infliction while wounds made through clothing suggest homicide.

The selection of certain areas may be indicative. Wounds directed towards the breasts and genitals are common in homicidal assaults, cuts of the wrists characteristic of suicide, while grouping of wounds

*References are to Bibliography beginning on page 159.

in the front of the neck or in the region of the heart may be seen in both types of case.

The presence of "defence" wounds consisting of cuts or bruises, usually located on the hands (Fig. 11-3) or forearms and sustained while fending off an assailant, would exclude suicide, but their absence does not eliminate homicide. When attempts to grasp the weapon have left cuts on the palm of the hand, their number and location may indicate whether the blade was single or double edged. "Hesitation cuts" which are superficial and usually multiple cuts in the immediate proximity of a lethal wound, are typical of suicidal injury.

The pathological examination of penetrating and incised wounds

All wounds should be numbered on the basis of a sketch or annotated photograph, and the distance of each from the nearest heel, the mid line and an anatomical landmark, such as the nipple or the umbilicus, measured. The shape and dimensions of each wound must be recorded, as well as the appearance of its edges, any undercutting, contusion or handle impression on the skin, the orientation of the blade and any sign of twisting or cutting.

The direction of all stab wounds and, if possible, their depth of penetration, should be determined. In the case of cuts the depth at each end of the wound should be ascertained.

Any injury, even of a trivial nature, on the fingers, hands or forearms must be described in detail. If there is any suggestion that the blade might have been broken, the body should be x-rayed and any blade fragments recovered.

The number and location of wounds on the body must be compared with any cuts in the clothing. Samples of blood for the determination of blood groups should be taken in all cases as well as samples of hair for comparison with any hairs which might be found on a suspect weapon.

12

FIREARM INJURIES

The number of injuries caused by firearms, both accidental and intentional, is directly related to the availability of such weapons in the community. Their frequency in North America is, therefore, amongst the highest in the world.

The large variety of weapons and ammunition makes this a difficult field in which the pathologist must rely on the firearms expert to a large extent. The subject of ballistics, which is concerned with the behaviour of projectiles, is generally divided into "internal" ballistics, which concerns the behaviour of the projectile within the weapon from which it is fired, "external" ballistics, its characteristics during flight, and "terminal" ballistics, its fate when striking or penetrating the target. Only the last phase, when the target has been the human body, falls within the realm of the pathological investigation.

In spite of his somewhat restricted role in the investigation of shooting fatalities the pathologist can contribute in a number of important respects. By a careful study of the injuries he may ascertain the number of shots fired, the distance and angle of firing, the type of weapon used and the feasibility of self infliction. By recovering the bullet and the securing of entrance wounds and the clothing he will aid in the identification of the actual weapon used. Unskilled or thoughtless work, on the other hand, can easily destroy important findings.

While there is an almost infinite variety of firearms, those encountered in practice belong to two general categories, those in which a single projectile is fired through a rifled barrel (rifles, revolvers, automatics) and those firing pellets or slugs through a smooth bore barrel. More rarely seen are injuries by air guns, rivet guns, guns firing a captive bolt which are used in the slaughtering of cattle, and the multiplicity of home made weapons ("zip guns") which may not only fire regular ammunition but also shoot marbles, nails and ball bearings.

Except in burned or decomposed bodies there is rarely any difficulty in the recognition of firearm injuries although certain types of stab wounds (Fig. 11-1) and electrical burns may simulate them. The wounds may, of course, be located in inconspicuous or concealed areas such as the arm pits, the ear canals or the inside of the mouth.

The determination of the number of shots depends on the correct identification of entrance ("inshoot") and exit ("outshoot") wounds and the findings of the projectiles in the body. It must be remembered that a bullet may fragment and produce two or more exit wounds and that a single projectile may transit a part of the body such as the neck or an arm and then re-enter causing several entrance wounds. The uncommon use of tandem ammunition in which two bullets are contained in the same round must also be kept in mind.

The mechanism of wounding

The extent of the destruction caused by a projectile is determined by the amount of energy delivered by it to the tissues. The initial kinetic energy with which the projectile strikes the body surface is a function of both its mass and its velocity. The amount of energy transferred to the tissues, however, depends not only on its initial energy but also on its rate of retardation in the tissue. The latter, in turn, depends on tissue density as well as on the shape and orientation of the projectile. It follows that, for a given initial kinetic energy, a bullet which leaves the body will have less wounding power than one which delivered its entire energy and thus remains in the tissue. Bullets which tumble or which undergo deformation such as soft or partially jacketed bullets are especially destructive.

Four mechanisms are concerned in the production of tissue injury:

(1) The transit of the missile. This is the only mechanism in low velocity missiles, less than 400 feet per second. The path of destruction is roughly of the same diameter as the projectile.

(2) Shock waves. In the case of a higher velocity projectile, the tissue ahead of it is compressed forming a circular shock wave which recedes from the projectile at the speed of sound. This causes relatively little tissue damage except to gas filled organs which may rupture.

(3) Temporary cavity. A projectile travelling in excess of 1000 feet per second transfers great energy to the tissue ahead of it and adjacent to its sides which thus moves away from its path even after the projectile has passed. This creates a cavity which has an "explosive" effect and causes extensive tissue disruption (Fig. 12-1). The size of the temporary cavity, which persists several milliseconds, is proportional to the energy delivered to the tissues.

(4) Permanent cavity. This is the defect which remains after the collapse of the temporary cavity. Its size depends mainly on

the size of the temporary cavity. Its diameter is always larger than that of the projectile except in the skin surface where, due to the elasticity of the skin, the diameter may be smaller. Tissue is lost internally by spilling into body cavities and externally by the "splash" which occurs at both entrance and exit wounds.

Other, less common, mechanisms of wounding include the effects of gas pressure in tight contact and of secondary missiles like pieces of the projectile, bone fragments or pieces of button.

Characteristics of bullet entrance and exit wounds

In the examination of a shooting victim the recognition of the wounds of entrance and exit is essential for the reconstruction of the event. At close range there is usually little difficulty as some of the

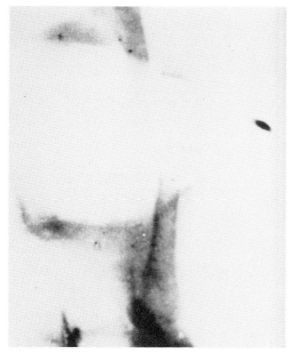

Fig. 12-1. X-ray of the thigh of a cat during the passage of a small shell fragment showing the large size of the temporary cavity compared with that of the projectile. (From Harvey et al.,[76] courtesy of the Surgeon General of the United States.)

features listed in Table 12-2 are likely to be present. The application of newer techniques, such as the detection of metal traces by neutron activation analysis, offers hope of extending the distance at which entrance wounds can be identified.[96]*

The microscopic examination of close range entrance wounds may show the scorching effect of the discharge gases[3] and traces of carbon monoxide have been demonstrated chemically.

At distances beyond two feet the surface changes are likely to be absent and the recognition of the entrance wounds becomes more difficult. Pieces of clothing, hairs etc. may be carried into the wound and, when bone is struck, bone fragments tend to be carried towards the exit wound. A projectile passing through a flat bone which has an outer and an inner layer, like the skull or the breast bone, leaves a characteristic cone shaped defect, the tip of the cone pointing towards the entrance.

The comparative sizes of entrance and exit wounds have received much study. Experimentally, when steel spheres are shot through animal tissue, the wound of exit is smaller than that of entrance because of the sphere's loss of energy during its passage.[99] In practice, however, the general rule that the exit wound is larger generally holds, because the size of the wound also depends on the orientation of the projectile as it enters or leaves the body. Bullets, unlike spheres, are likely to yaw or to become deformed, thus producing a larger exit defect. The most common exceptions are entrance wounds with tight contact discharges over bone and those due to ricochets which are usually larger than the exit wounds. High velocity projectiles passing through soft tissue only may produce entrance and exit wounds of equal size.

The feasibility of suicide

Investigating the circumstances of a shooting, whether suicidal, accidental or homicidal, is a matter for the police. The pathologist will, nevertheless, often be asked about the possibility of self infliction.

While in accidents or suicides the firing distance will generally be within the reach of the victim and the entrance wound in an area accessible to him, it must be remembered that considerable ingenuity may be employed in triggering the weapon (by a toe, string or stick), particularly if it was intended to simulate an accident.

Contact wounds of the temples, the forehead, the front of the chest and shots into the mouth are nearly always self inflicted. Shots into the left side of the head by a right handed individual, shots through clothing, multiple shots and the absence of cadaveric rigidity of the hands do not exclude suicide.

---

*References are to Bibliography beginning on page 159.

Table 12-2
The surface characteristics of close range entrance wounds

Surface characteristic	Synonyms	Cause	Comments
Skin defect	Permanent cavity	Bullet, slug	Often smaller than diameter of projectile, may contain textile fibers, hairs and, in very close range wounds, powder grains
		Shot pellets	Appearance of defect(s) depends on type of ammunition, distance and barrel choke
		Wad	Penetration of skin rare at distances over 6 feet
Abraded margin	Contusion ring	Projectile	Independent of firing distance, may be absent over bone (skull)
Radiating tears		Gas	Tight contact over bone
Gray ring	Contact ring	Lead of bullet lubricant	Independent of firing distance, may be absent with jacketed bullets or obscured by abraded margin
Muzzle impression	Muzzle contusion	Muzzle of weapon	Contact or near contact, skin pressed against muzzle by gas or by temporary cavity
Smudging	Blackening, fouling	Partially burned gases	Close range, more marked with black powder, may be absent under clothing and in tight contact wounds
Tattooing	Stippling	Powder grains	Close range, more marked with black powder, may be absent under clothing or in tight contact wounds
Singeing	Burning	Hot gases	Close range, more marked with black powder, in tight contact wounds the deeper tissues may show heat effects

Testing for nitrate residues on the hands of the victim (paraffin test, Gonzales test) has been largely abandoned because of lack of specificity,[34] but traces of blood or brain tissue on the hands or on the muzzle of the weapon may be very important.

The nature of the muzzle discharge

Apart from the projectile itself, many other materials are expelled from the muzzle during the discharge of a firearm. Some of these, like gases, may play a part in wound production, while others may be deposited in or around the entrance wound. These materials include unburned or partially burned powder grains (Fig. 12-4), carbon particles, traces of bullet lubricant (grease, wax), traces of primer components (lead, barium, nitrates), fragments of soft bullets (lead, antimony), fragments of bullet jackets (copper, nickel) and metal traces

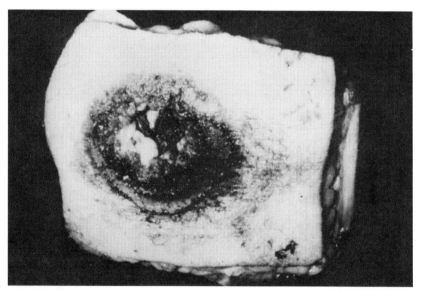

Fig. 12-3. Close range entrance wound excised for submission to the laboratory.

derived from the cartridge case or the barrel. The greater the density of such particles and the greater their energy, the longer their travelling distance (Fig. 12-5).

When the sealing of powder gases between the cartridge case and the firing chamber or between the bullet and the barrel (obturation) is poor, gas leakage will occur and gases will precede the bullet from the muzzle. Such deficient obturation would also reduce the velocity of the projectile.

In the case of shotgun ammunition, materials expelled, apart from the pellets or slug, also include crimps, wads and fragments of the shell.

The pathological examination of rifle and handgun injuries

After the body has been photographed, the clothing is removed and each item showing a bullet hole put into a separate container. If it is necessary to cut the clothing, the cuts must avoid the bullet holes. The clothing must not be allowed to fall on the floor and care must be taken to detect loose bullets.

After the body has been undressed, it is photographed again. The location of all bullet wounds should be described in relation to anatomical landmarks (nipples, umbilicus) and the distance from the nearest heel measured. Probes may be useful in demonstrating the direction of the path of bullets but the creating of artificial tracks by excessive force must, of course, be avoided.

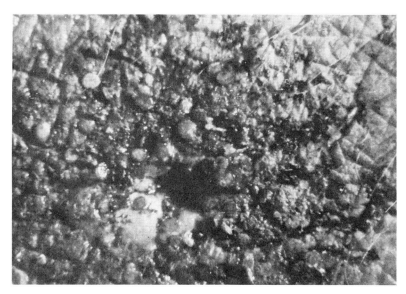

Fig. 12-4. Appearance under a magnifying glass of the entrance wound made by a .22 caliber bullet fired at close range. Surrounding the wound is an irregular area in which the skin has been denuded (abraded margin). Outside this are areas of blackening and unburned powder grains in the form of round discs.

Close-up photographs, which include a scale, should be taken of each wound. Washing of wounds, while making the recognition of entrance wounds easier and improving their photographic appearance, is not recommended as it tends to remove surface deposits.

Fluoroscopy is helpful in locating elusive bullets, and x-ray plates serve as permanent records and are the best means of studying the distribution of bullet or bone fragments.

Close range entrance wounds should be excised together with the surrounding skin and deeper tissues (Fig. 12-3). These should not be washed but gentle immersion in fixative is permissible.

As much as possible of the projectile should be submitted for examination. Soft bullets will often be intact although deformed, while partially jacketed bullets may have separated into the soft core and the jacket. Handling bullets with metal instruments should be avoided and no identifying marks (initials, numbers) should be scratched on them. The bullets should not be washed as hairs or textile fibers may be adherent to them. When the projectile has greatly fragmented, the fragments may have to be recovered by macerating or chemically digesting the tissue.

All bullets or bullet fragments should be put into separate containers which are sealed and initialled.

Shotgun injuries

The surface configuration of shotgun entrance wounds, except those due to a single ball or slug, enables the examiner to estimate the firing distance over a much greater range than in the case of bullet wounds. The actual determination, however, should be left to the firearms expert, as it involves the reconstruction of the shooting by using the actual gun with the proper type of ammunition and degree of choke.

The width of scatter of the pellets depends on the distance and choke, not on their size. The density of the pattern, on the other hand, reflects the number of pellets in the shell and thus "the smaller the shot, the denser the pattern". As each pellet has a relatively low kinetic energy, exit wounds of the trunk are not often seen. The wounding power of wads is small but their recovery will help in the identification of the type of ammunition and its manufacturer.

Although the degree of barrel choke, which is one of the variables affecting the scatter of shot pellets, is usually not known, the following appearances provide an initial estimate of the firing distance.

The entrance wound up to a distance of one foot will be a single round hole with sharp edges and considerable blackening and powder deposits on the surrounding surface. Up to a distance of three feet the wound may remain a single defect although scalloping of the edges becomes noticeable and the blackening and powder deposits less marked. At distances up to three feet the wads are likely to be found in the wound. At a distance of six feet a large central defect is usually still present but is surrounded by a few pellet holes. The wads at that distance tend to cause a separate injury but do not often penetrate the skin, merely producing a small contusion. At 12 feet the separation of pellets is complete and the wads do not reach the body surface. At 30 feet the field of scatter is so great that not all the pellets strike the body.

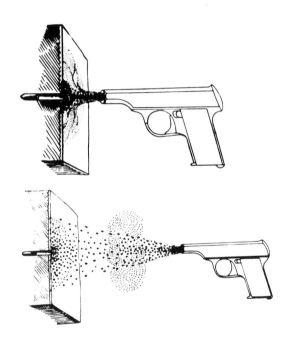

Fig. 12-5. From the deposits surrounding a close range entrance wound, the firing distance may be deduced, provided the same weapon and ammunition are used in test firing. (From Ponsold.[142] By permission, The Georg Thieme Company.)

Additional steps in the examination of shotgun injuries

The field of scatter is measured both vertically and horizontally, disregarding any greatly eccentric pellets ("flyers").

X-ray plates show well the distribution of pellets in the tissues (Fig. 12-6) but measurements of the field of scatter from x-rays are likely to be erroneous because of parallax.

All wads and as many pellets as possible should be submitted to the laboratory.

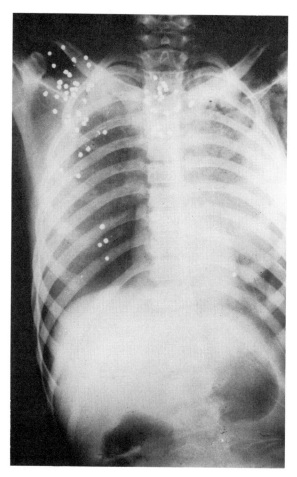

Fig. 12-6. The distribution of shotgun pellets in the body can be studied only by means of x-rays.

13

SKELETAL REMAINS

The discovery of skeletons is common during the summer months when highway and building construction are at their peak and when the commercial operation of sand and gravel pits uncovers old burial grounds. In the autumn the hunting season regularly yields, apart from slaughtered deer, the remnants of lost and hunted hunters.

Bones are also occasionally found during the demolition of old houses and, while the possibility of crime must never be forgotten, the pathologist may avoid embarrassment by considering the possibility that these may be old anatomical specimens. Good preservation of muscles and tendons in obviously old specimens, the presence of saw cuts or signs of bleaching or varnishing should alert him. Occasionally the finding of screws or hinges will add a welcome note of reassurance.

The detailed study of skeletal remains is likely to lead into special fields in which the pathologist would be wise to call on the help of other experts, but even a preliminary inspection may answer many questions. The information to be gained by the examination of skeletons is necessarily limited by the absence of the body surface and the internal organs. On the other hand, injuries to bone, such as bullet wounds or skull fractures, may remain recognisable for decades and by their nature and location indicate the existence of certain internal injuries.

The identification of skeletal remains

Age. Childhood, puberty and adolescence are periods of rapid skeletal development and it is not surprising that they provide more precise indicators of age than the long periods of maturity and senescence which follow. The skeleton of the fetus initially consists entirely of membrane or cartilage but from the sixth week of intra-uterine life onwards develops small islands of bone (centres of ossification) in an orderly sequence and distribution. These become more numerous and larger until the age of 20 years.

The ends of the long bones (epiphyses) are separated from the shafts until the age of 15 years but then gradually unite with them. This union or fusion of epiphyses also occurs in a known sequence and continues until the 26th year.

Both the appearance of the centres of ossification and the fusion of epiphyses can be followed by x-ray and provide the most accurate index of age but it must be remembered that females tend to precede males by as much as two years by puberty.[91, 96, 117*]

The changes in the skull, again, are precise indicators of age only in the early age period. Two soft spots (fontanelles) are present at the time of birth, the posterior one closing at the age of 8 weeks, the anterior one at 18 months. The gradual disappearance of the sutures of the skull during adult life has acquired an undeserved reputation for accuracy. It is so variable that, at best, it can be regarded as an indicator of the decade.

Changes in the joint surface of the pubic bone have recently been studied because these provide the only guide during early adult life, which is a period otherwise devoid of conspicuous changes.[117] At the age of 17 to 18 years this joint surface has a series of transverse ridges and grooves ("billowing") which gradually become obliterated thus roughly indicating the age (Fig. 13-1).

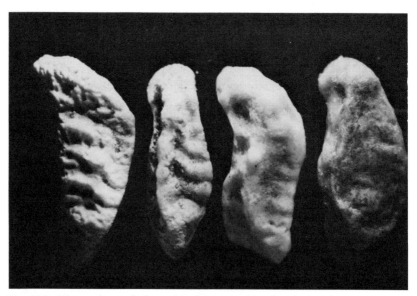

Fig. 13-1. The surfaces of the pubic joint of white female individuals ages (left to right) 19, 26, 33 and 41 years showing the gradual disappearance of transverse ridges.

---

*References are to Bibliography beginning on page 159.

Senile changes. It is understandable that no consistent chronological incidence can be expected of changes which are essentially pathological in nature. These include calcification of the rib and laryngeal cartilages, arthritic changes in joints and rarification of bones. These are rarely marked before the age of 40 but increase both in frequency and severity in the subsequent decades.

Race. The determination of race is difficult even for the expert and is largely based on a number of skull measurements and their ratios and the proportion of limb to trunk lengths. The assignment of the remains to the Caucasoid, Negroid or Mongoloid (Chinese, Japanese, North American Indian) racial groups is the most that can be accomplished, even with the help of a physical anthropologist. If hair is also found it may help to establish the racial origin.

Sex. Most sexual characteristics of the skeleton appear after puberty making the sexing of mature skeletons relatively simple. According to Krogman[96] sex could be determined with 100 per cent accuracy if the entire skeleton was available, with 95 per cent accuracy on the basis of the pelvic bone alone and with 90 per cent accuracy by the skull alone.

Generally, the bones of females are more slender with less prominent markings for muscle attachments. Their limbs are shorter in relation to the trunk and the width of the shoulders is less or equal to the width of the hip. The skull, pelvis, spine, breast bone and the thigh bone are the parts of the skeleton upon which the determination of sex is based.

Stature. The estimate of body stature forms part of the examination of every unidentified skeleton. In comparing the findings with the living heights of persons it must be remembered that the latter are often estimates rather than measurements and that, even if measurements, they may have been made many years before death.

Direct measurements, even of complete skeletons are not sufficiently accurate because they involve making allowance for skin, soft tissues, intervertebral discs and spinal curvature.

Body height is thus determined indirectly by measuring individual long bones. During the past 50 years many tables showing the relation of long bone measurements to body height have been published. These tables, however, have been based on the studies of certain populations and, as the relation of bone length to body length is both a sex and a racial characteristic, such data must be used with great caution. The old rule: "length of arm bone (humerus) x 5 = body length" is not sufficiently accurate for forensic purposes.

In the specific phase of the identification, abnormalities of the skeleton, such as old fractures, are of obvious importance but, as has been pointed out, this phase of the identification depends on the existence of pre mortem records of such abnormalities.

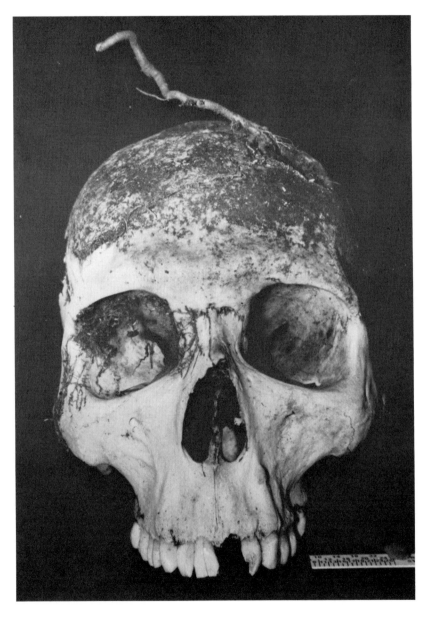

Fig. 13-2. Male skull found in the bush. The cedar root growing through a bullet exit wound on the left side was found to be six years old, thus giving a minimum age to the specimen.

X-ray examination may be very helpful, especially when studying bone fragments. Most bones of the body consist of a hard shell (cortex) which surrounds a cavity. The latter is filled with a spongy mass of small bone spicules (trabeculae) the pattern of which, as shown by x-ray, is as distinctive as a fingerprint. In addition, the cortex is penetrated by blood vessels, the number and location of which vary from individual to individual. Although the blood vessels themselves are no longer present, the small channels in which they had been located are easily visible on x-ray and constitute another individual peculiarity.

How old are the remains?

The dating of skeletal remains is difficult because the changes which occur in the bony matrix are determined by the physical and chemical conditions of the environment in which they had been lying, particularly with regard to moisture and acidity, rather than by the time elapsed since death. The persistence for centuries of skeletons in dry vaults on the one hand, and their rapid demineralization in acid ground on the other, are familiar examples.

Estimates of bone age are based upon the presence of remnants of soft tissue, the persistence of tissue protein (precipitin reaction, nitrogen content, amino acids), collagen (fluorescence under ultraviolet light, the content of proline and hydroxyproline) or hemoglobin (benzidine test), their consistency (replacement of phosphates by carbonates or silicates) and the demonstration of fat or fatty acids (adipocere).

Generally, the pathologist will be able to decide without much difficulty whether the remains are more than 50 years old and thus likely to be of mere historical or archaeological interest, or of more recent origin and possibly of forensic significance. Beyond this, any estimate must remain a rough approximation.

Additional clues to the age of remains may be derived from the presence of permeating plant roots (Fig. 13-2) and artefacts such as nails, pottery, fragments of coffin and, in the case of Indian remains, beads, ornaments and weapons.

As the large number and variety of tests shown in the following table indicates, a reliable method of dating skeletal remains still has to be found. The times shown in the table indicate maximum "lying times".

"Lying times" of skeletal remains

Less than 50 years:

    Remnants of clothing (textiles, leather) — 5 years.
    Positive benzidine test — 10 years.

Positive precipitin test for human protein — 15 years.
Remnants of desiccated muscle and tendons — 10 to 20 years.
Demonstrable fat — 10 years.
Demonstrable fatty acids — 20 years.
Diffuse strong fluorescence under ultraviolet light — 50 years.
Normal consistency — 50 years.
Nitrogen content more that 3.5 grams per cent — 50 years.

More than 50 years:

Increased fragility.
Replacement of phosphate by carbonate and silicate.
Weak and patchy fluorescence under ultraviolet light.
Absence of proline and hydroxyproline.
Less than 7 amino acids demonstrable.[94]

14

THE EMBALMED BODY, EXHUMATIONS

The embalmed body

The various methods of embalming, some of which originated in remotest history, have as their objective the preservation of the body by the prevention of autolysis and putrefaction. Embalming was a common practice and one of great religious significance amongst the ancient Egyptians, reaching its peak during the 22nd dynasty (950 to 730 B.C.) but continuing for several centuries into the Christian era. It also seems to have been practised in some of the South and Central American civilizations, particularly by the Incas.

In Europe during the Middle Ages the practice fell into disuse, but this period provided interesting instances of natural embalming in the form of bodies buried in the acid soil of swamps and marshes ("bog people"). Many such bodies, originating from the tenth, eleventh and twelfth centuries and some extremely well preserved, have now been found, mostly in Denmark but also in Holland, England, Scotland and northern Germany.[59]*

The modern practice of embalming received its impetus during the American Civil War when it made possible the transportation of the Union war dead to their home states, and the majority of the dead in North America are now embalmed. The practice is less common in Great Britain and even less so in continental Europe. While the primary objective of modern embalming is still preservation, secondary objectives are the restoration of a "life-like" appearance and the destruction of hazardous bacteria. In many countries embalming is now obligatory whenever bodies must be transported over long distances or when burial or cremation must be delayed.

Modern embalming usually employs one or more of the following techniques:

(1) The perfusion under pressure of the arterial system with approximately 3 gallons (11 to 12 litres) of a fixative embalm-

*References are to Bibliography beginning on page 159.

ing fluid and the simultaneous drainage of blood from the venous side of the circulation.

(2) The instillation of "cavity fluid" into the body cavities by means of a trocar, usually introduced through the abdominal wall.

(3) The hypodermic injection of embalming fluid into regions not adequately fixed by the perfusion technique.

(4) The local application of embalming fluid or powders to organs in autopsied cases and to external lesions such as ulcers or wounds.

In addition, many materials are applied to the skin to conceal incisions, to retard drying and for cosmetic purposes.[168]

Embalming materials comprise a large variety of chemical substances, the most common being ethyl and methyl alcohol, isopropyl alcohol, formaldehyde ("formalin"), paraformaldehyde, phenol, para-dichlorobenzene, ethylene glycol, glycerol, potassium nitrate, benzoic acid and pyidine, in addition to various dyes and perfumes. The latter include methyl salicylate ("oil of wintergreen").

Most provinces of Canada and states of the United States have statutory requirements concerning the composition of embalming materials. These usually specify the percentage of formaldehyde in the various fluids and many prohibit the use of arsenic or salts of heavy metals (mercury, lead, zinc) as well as that of alkaloids like strychnine.

The autopsy on embalmed bodies

As far as the pathologist is concerned, embalming is a mixed blessing. He is not likely to be misled by the embalming incisions or trocar marks but the subcutaneous injection of fluids or filling materials and the external application of powders and cosmetics may mask lesions. The organs are likely to have been disrupted by the trocar and the contents of the gastro-intestinal tract spilled into the abdominal cavity. Thrombi may have been dissolved and the isolation of bacteria is no longer feasible.

In view of the multiplicity of chemical substances in embalming materials and the large volume of embalming fluids employed, it is understandable that the task of the toxicologist is made more difficult, especially as far as quantitative determinations are concerned. The qualitative detection, however, of many common drugs and poisons, such as barbiturates, carbon monoxide, strychnine and heavy metals, remains largely unaffected.

The ethyl alcohol content of many embalming fluids precludes any meaningful analysis for this substance in blood and tissues, although recently analysis of the fluid in the eye ball (vitreous humour) has been found to reveal alcohol levels similar to those found in the blood before embalming.[155]

Whenever toxicological analysis is indicated, tissue specimens should be taken from the least well fixed parts of organs. If possible, samples of the embalming materials used should be obtained from the undertaker and also submitted.

While toxicological analysis is complicated by the embalming process, signs of physical injury are preserved for a long time. An embalmed body, therefore, offers a much greater scope for pathological examination than a decomposed one, a great advantage especially after long periods of burial.

Exhumations

Strictly, the term "exhumation" denotes the recovery of any buried body, but in general usage refers to the disinterment of a body from a grave in a cemetery or burial ground. The authority for such an exhumation is issued by a coroner, judge, district or crown attorney under an appropriate piece of legislation.[90]

Exhumations are carried out either for the purpose of transporting a body to another burial site, a procedure which usually does not involve the pathologist, or for medical examination. The aim of the latter may be the verification of the deceased's identity, or the determination of the cause of death or both.

As an exhumation often involves the recovery of a certain body from an area in which perhaps thousands of other bodies are buried, the identity of the body assumes great importance, particularly in cases of criminal prosecution.

Exhumation procedure

The pathologist should be present during the entire procedure. Before being opened, the burial plot should be identified by a cemetery official on the basis of the cemetery register. The name of the deceased on the grave stone is not sufficient.

Any vault should then be identified by the person who supplied it, usually the undertaker. Vaults may bear the name of the deceased but should be identified at least as to type.

After having been raised and before being opened, the coffin should be identified by the undertaker, at least as to type and make.

After the opening of the coffin the body itself is identified. If visual identification is not possible because of post mortem changes, the identification may have to be based on articles of clothing or jewellery. The body should be removed from the coffin for examination.

In the recovery of any buried body, samples of soil should be collected in clean glass containers and their precise origin in relation to the body recorded. Samples should also be obtained of material found within the coffin such as fabric of coffin lining, soil and water. The results of any toxicological analysis of tissue can be properly interpreted only in the light of the findings in these samples.

15

THE "NEGATIVE" AUTOPSY

It seems reasonable to expect that functional disturbance, severe enough to have caused death, would always be reflected in structural alteration which could be demonstrated post mortem, and this expectation is largely borne out by the experience with hospital autopsies. In forensic practice, however, the pathologist frequently encounters instances in which no cause of death can be demonstrated either anatomically or by toxicological analysis.

The suspicion naturally arises that a significant lesion may have been missed, a possibility which can, of course, never be entirely excluded. The temptation is then great to attribute excessive importance to minor or equivocal findings, particularly if the pathologist is under pressure to produce an acceptable diagnosis. The ultimate interests of justice and medicine, however, are better served by leaving the diagnosis open than by attaching a spurious label. The wiser and the more experienced the pathologist, therefore, the greater his reluctance to attribute death to minor lesions and the higher his proportion of inconclusive cases. In the experience of most pathologists 5 to 10 per cent of their cases fall into this category.

In the absence of diagnostic pathological findings, much may have to be inferred from the circumstances under which death occurred and from the medical history of the deceased. Death from status asthmaticus, for instance, has no diagnostic findings but evidence of asthma may be seen in the lungs and a history of asthmatic attacks may be obtained. The same applies to death from status epilepticus in epileptic individuals. In the absence of clinical information any medication or prescriptions found amongst the personal effects may become very important. It is essential to bear in mind, as has been pointed out in previous chapters, that an expected cause of death may not have been the cause of death.

Post mortem decomposition and the destruction by insects and animals progressively increase the number of "negative" cases by obscuring bruises and by distorting or obliterating lacerations, so that, as the body approaches skeletonization, all signs of soft tissue injury disappear. The number of inconclusive cases thus bears a direct relationship to the degree of body destruction.

The following are some relatively common conditions in which the pathological findings, even in well preserved bodies, will be suggestive rather than diagnostic or in which the examination will fail to reveal any significant abnormalities at all.

Vagal inhibition. The two vagus nerves arise from the brain stem and, after having passed through the neck, one on each side, enter the chest and supply branches to the heart muscle. The normal action of the vagus nerves slows the heart beat, but abnormally strong stimulation may stop heart action completely. These nerves may be stimulated directly by pressure on the sides of the neck and instances of even slight pressure producing sudden cardiac arrest are known to every forensic pathologist (Fig. 9-2).

Indirect stimulation is more common and may be triggered by a large variety of surgical procedures and minor injuries, many surprisingly trivial. They include needle punctures, dilatation of body sphincters, stripping of adhesive tape from the skin and manipulation of the nose and larynx. Death following the sudden immersion into cold water ("immersion syndrome") also seems to be an instance of vagal inhibition[161]* and the mechanism has been suspected in the "crib death" of infants.

There are no diagnostic autopsy findings so that the diagnosis is one of exclusion.

Exposure (hypothermia). A body temperature of 34°C (93.2°F) cannot be tolerated for long and a body temperature of 30°C (86°F) rapidly causes death by interfering with heart action. Death from exposure is seen in abandoned infants, in elderly and debilitated persons, and in lost hunters, mountain climbers and occupants of life boats. The ingestion of alcohol accelerates heat loss by dilating the blood vessels of the skin. Autopsy findings are not specific and include ulcers of the stomach and intestine and lesions of the pancreas.[108, 182]

Heat stroke (hyperthermia). In persons exposed to a source of heat an intolerably high body temperature may develop if the body's temperature regulating mechanisms break down. The findings are not diagnostic and the lesions of the liver and brain which have been described[63, 106] are probably due to terminal shock rather than to the high temperature per se.

Drug reaction. Some fatal reactions to drugs appear to involve an allergic mechanism and cause airway obstruction by swelling of the larynx. Other reactions, however, to which the name "idiosyncrasy" is

---

*References are to Bibliography beginning on page 159.

often applied, involve an unknown mechanism and have no diagnostic post mortem findings.

Poisonings. The toxicological analysis may be inconclusive when unstable substances such as chloral hydrate or very volatile agents are involved, or when the survival time has been long enough to have permitted the elimination of the poison.

Electrocution. Unlike deaths due to lightning or industrial electrocution which usually show burns of various degrees of severity, those occurring in the home, particularly in the bath or swimming pool, may show no burns or internal lesions.

Insulin overdose (hypoglycemia). There are generally no findings but a history of insulin medication may be obtained. If recent needle marks are present they should be excised and analyzed. The hormone has been detected in needle marks in a homicide by insulin injection[18] and in bile in a case of suicide by insulin.[169]

Breathing of an inert gas. Upon entering an atmosphere of a nonrespirable gas such as methane or nitrogen, which is not an uncommon industrial mishap, death occurs very quickly and there are no pathological findings apart from scattered petechial hemorrhages.

The difficulties inherent in the recognition of drowning and smothering and of "crib deaths" are discussed in the appropriate chapters.

A diagnosis by exclusion or by inference is never satisfying but, in spite of their understandable reluctance, police officers, coroners and the courts must accept the fact that this is often the best that can be accomplished.

This group of indeterminate cases represents, in a sense, the scientific frontier of forensic pathology. The largely unexplored applications of electron microscopy, trace analysis, virology and histochemistry to medico-legal problems offer fascinating prospects of a better understanding of these conditions and of new and more specific diagnostic tools.

.

GLOSSARY OF SOME TERMS
USED IN FORENSIC MEDICINE

Abortifacient: A substance or instrument used to procure an *abortion* by causing the death of the fetus or by stimulating uterine contractions which result in the expulsion of the fetus.

Abortion: 1. The expulsion of the fetus, usually in the first trimester of pregnancy.
2. The interruption of pregnancy before the age of fetal viability.

Abraded margin: Syn. abrasion collar, marginal abrasion. A zone of abrasion surrounding the entrance wound of a bullet, caused by the stretching of the skin and the rotational movement of the projectile.

Abrasion collar: *See* abraded margin.

Abscess: An area of tissue destruction containing pus.

Acid phosphatase: A group of enzymes occurring in many cells of the body. The only secretion in which acid phosphatase is found in significant concentration is that of the prostate gland. The detection of acid phosphatase in more than trace amounts in vaginal washings or on clothing is thus regarded as indicating the presence of seminal fluid.

Activation analysis: Syn. neutron activation, radio activation. An analytical method for the detection of trace elements in biological materials. Irradiation by nuclear particles induces radioactivity in these elements which can then be detected by their characteristic emissions. The forensic applications of activation analysis include the analysis of hairs and nails, the examination of bullet entrance areas for the determination of the firing distance and the establishment of the individuality of hairs.

Addiction: A severe psychological and physical dependence on a drug such as alcohol or a narcotic. Sudden abstinence from the drug will result in withdrawal symptoms.

Adipocire: Syn. adipocere. A waxy greyish-white substance consisting largely of free fatty acids, produced by the hydrolysis of body fat in a moist environment. See also Table 1-6.

Agonal: Adj. Related to the last moments of life or to the death struggle.

Air embolism: *See* embolism.

Alcohol: A hydroxy derivative of aliphatic hydrocarbons. When used without qualification the term denotes ethyl alcohol, syn.

ethanol, grain alcohol, the active constituent of alcoholic beverages. Alcohols are central nervous system depressants.

methyl alcohol: Syn. methanol, wood alcohol. A common industrial solvent and constituent of resins and varnishes. It is much more toxic than ethyl alcohol.

Alcohol dehydrogenase: Syn. L.A.D.H. A zinc containing ferment in the liver catalyzing the early stages in the oxidation of ethyl alcohol and some of the higher alcohols.

Amniotic fluid: Syn. liquor amnii. The liquid in the amniotic sac in which the fetus is suspended. It contains cells of the fetal skin and *lanugo hairs*. It is usually clear or slightly milky but may contain blood, bile or meconium (*see* meconium). Entrance of amniotic fluid into the maternal veins causes amniotic fluid embolism (*see* embolism).

Amniotic fluid embolism: See embolism.

Amphetamines: Syn. "speed". A group of drugs which includes amphetamine sulphate, methylamphetamine and dextroamphetamine. The amphetamines are central nervous system stimulants which in therapeutic doses cause elevation of mood, alertness, increase in mental ability and reduction of appetite. In toxic doses they cause restlessness, irritability, hallucinations and panic states. Brain hemorrhage may be a terminal event.

Analgesic: A drug relieving pain.

Anaphylaxis: An acute and sometimes fatal reaction occurring within seconds or minutes after exposure to an allergen to which an individual is hypersensitive.

Aneurysm: A localized bulging of a blood vessel or chamber of the heart arising in a weakness of its wall.

arterio-venous aneurysm: An aneurysm involving a direct communication between an artery and a vein. Arterio-venous aneurysms may be congenital in origin or be caused by an injury.

berry aneurysm: Syn. congenital aneurysm. An aneurysm involving one of the arteries at the base of the brain. Rupture of a berry aneurysm is a common cause of sudden death in young or middle aged adults.

dissecting aneurysm: A diffuse swelling of an artery caused by the penetration of blood between the various layers of the vessel wall.

fusiform aneurysm: A spindle shaped dilatation of a blood vessel involving its entire circumference.

mycotic aneurysm: An aneurysm arising in a weakness of a blood vessel wall caused by infection.

saccular aneurysm: A sac-like aneurysm arising in a localized weakness of the vessel wall, involving only a portion of the circumference and connected to the lumen of the vessel by a narrower neck.

traumatic aneurysm: An aneurysm arising from a point of blood vessel injury.

Anoxia: A complete lack of oxygen.

Ante mortem: Adj. Syn. pre mortem. Present or occurring before death.

Anterior: Adj. Syn. ventral. Before, in front of, facing towards the front.

Anthropometry: The measurement of certain bodily features

such as standing height, arm reach, head diameters etc., introduced by Bertillon in 1882 as an aid in the identification of individuals.

Anthropophagy: The eating of a human body by animals.

Antimony: A poisonous metallic element in common industrial use. Its medicinal use is now confined to a few preparations employed in tropical medicine. The metal is also a component of soft bullets and of the core of jacketed bullets.

Aorta: The main artery arising from the heart and giving rise to the entire systemic arterial system.

Arachnoid mater: The middle membrane covering the brain and spinal cord.

Arsenic: A poisonous element and a common constituent of weed killers, insecticides and rat killers. Formerly widely used in medicine.

Artefact: Syn. artifact. A change brought about artificially and not by natural processes.

Arteriosclerosis: A group of pathological conditions affecting arteries and resulting in hardening, thickening and loss of elasticity of the wall and often in narrowing of the lumen.

Artery: A blood vessel carrying blood on its way from the heart to the tissues of the body.

coronary artery: One of two arteries arising from the *aorta* and supplying the heart.

Asphyxia: Death caused by lack of oxygen or by the inability of the tissues to use oxygen.

traumatic asphyxia: Asphyxia produced by compression of the chest and prevention of respiratory movements. Common in industrial accidents.

Atheroma: A localized form of *arteriosclerosis* consisting of a focal proliferation of fibrous tissue and the deposition of fats, and resulting in a narrowing of the lumen. Atheroma commonly involves the coronary arteries and the arteries of the brain.

Autoeroticism: Sexual gratification without a partner.

Autolysis: The dissolution of cells and tissues by enzymes normally present in them. Autolysis is the earliest structural post mortem change and is the predominant change in sterile cadavers such as newborn infants. It is also the main mechanism in the dissolution of infarcts (*see* infarct).

Automatism: A state in which a subject may perform actions without conscious volition or purpose. A state of automatism may follow brain injuries or epileptic seizures.

Autopsy: Syn. necropsy, postmortem. A dissection of the body after death to determine the cause of death, sometimes the identity of the deceased and to study the changes in the tissues caused by disease or violence. The term is often used to include any subsequent microscopic or chemical examination.

Azoospermia: The complete absence of sperm cells (spermatozoa) from the semen.

"Bag": Syn. "deck". A container of drugs.

"Bag man": Syn. "connection", "dealer", "mother", "pusher", "swing man". A supplier of illicit drugs.

Ballistics: The study of the behaviour of projectiles.

external ballistics: The behaviour of projectiles in flight.

internal ballistics: The behaviour of projectiles within the weapon from which they were fired.

terminal ballistics: The behaviour of projectiles when striking the target.

wound ballistics: The mechanism of wound production by projectiles.

Barbiturates: Syn. "barbs", "candy", "goof balls". A group of drugs used as *sedatives*, hypnotics and anaesthetics. They include thiopental (ultra-short acting), pentobarbital and secobarbital (short acting), amobarbital (intermediate) and phenobarbital (long acting).

Barotrauma: Injuries, such as rupture of the ear drum, caused by sudden change in atmospheric pressure.

Barrel: The tubular portion of a firearm through which the projectile passes.

Bends: *See* caisson disease.

Benzedrine: Brand of amphetamine sulphate (Smith, Kline and French Laboratories) Benzedrine tablets syn. "bennies", "hearts", "peaches", "roses".

Benzidine test: A test for the presence of hemoglobin.

Berry aneurysm: *See* aneurysm.

Bestiality: Sexual intercourse with an animal.

Birth injury: Syn. birth trauma. An injury to the infant sustained during birth. Common birth injuries include fractures of the skull, rupture of the venous sinuses of the dura, brain damage, stretching of nerves and dislocation of joints.

Blister: Syn. bleb, bulla, vesicle. An elevation of the superficial layer of the skin or mucous membrane containing fluid. When small often called a bleb or vesicle, when large a bulla. Blisters may be pre mortem or post mortem in origin.

Blood groups: Individuals who have the same type of blood with regard to the two red cell antigens A and B. Persons having antigen A only are said to be blood group A, those possessing antigen B only, blood group B, those having both antigens blood group AB and those having neither antigen blood group O.

"Blue velvet": Blue tablets of tripelennamine (pyribenzamine — Ciba), an antihistamine. They are often combined with a narcotic such as paregoric. When used intravenously lung lesions are produced (*see* "junkie's lung").

Bolus: A rounded and moistened mass of food ready for swallowing.

Bone marrow embolism: *See* embolism.

Bore: The inside of a firearm barrel.

bore diameter: *See* caliber.

Brandhematom: An extradural collection of brick red, friable blood clot in bodies which had been exposed to intense heat. Differentiation from pre mortem extradural hematoma may be difficult. The absence of skull fractures and a high carbon monoxide content of the clot favour brandhematom.

Bruise: A hemorrhage into the tissues beneath the skin. Bruises are usually caused by violence but may be spontaneous in certain disorders of the blood. During life the colour of bruises changes gradually, giving a rough indication of their ages.

Buck shot: Shotgun pellets having a diameter of more than .22 inches (9 to 12 pellets per shell).

Bulla: A large blister.

Bullet: A projectile fired from a rifled weapon (*see* rifle). Bullets may be soft (lead) or jacketed.

bullet embolism: *See* embolism

Burke: William (1792-1829). Executed in Edinburgh, Scotland, for having, in collaboration with William Hare and Helen Dougal, murdered about 15 persons for the purpose of selling their bodies for anatomical dissection.

"Burking": A homicidal form of traumatic *asphyxia* employed by Burke and Hare in which one of the assailants sat on the victim's chest.

Burn: An injury caused by dry heat.

"Burn": Purchasing an inferior or substituted illicit drug.

Cadaver: A dead body, a corpse.

Cadaveric: Adj. Pertaining to or belonging to a dead body.

cadaveric rigidity: *See* rigor mortis (Table 1-3).

cadaveric spasm: *See* rigor mortis (Table 1-3).

"Cafe coronary": Asphyxia due to the impaction of a bolus of food in the larynx or windpipe.

Caisson disease: Syn. decompression sickness, "the bends". A form of gas embolism (*see* embolism) seen in divers, tunnel workers etc. who are being brought quickly from an environment of high atmospheric pressure to one of lower pressure. It is caused by the release of bubbles of nitrogen from the blood.

Caliber: The inside diameter of the barrel of a firearm. In rifled barrels it is the distance from land to land (*see* lands).

Calliphora vomitoria: Syn. blow fly, blue bottle fly. A common fly which deposits its eggs upon recently dead bodies and the larvae of which play an important role in the disintegration of the tissues.

Callus: The tissues which gradually connect the fragments of a broken bone. Callus at first consists of fibrous tissue which is later converted into bone. The microscopic and x-ray appearance of a callus is roughly indicative of its age and thus may often be of importance in cases of suspected battered child syndrome.

"Candy": Cocaine.

"Candy man": A seller of cocaine.

Cantharides: Syn. "Spanish fly". The active component of the extract of the tissues of the blister beetle (Cantharis vesicatoria) which is wrongly regarded as having aphrodisiac properties but which may cause severe kidney damage.

"Cap": A capsule, a quantity of a drug such as heroin, cocaine or morphine.

Carbon monoxide: A toxic gas produced by the incomplete combustion of organic materials. It combines with hemoglobin, thus preventing the carriage of oxygen, and producing a state of asphyxia. Carbon monoxide is an important constituent of motor exhaust gas and coal gas.

Carbon tetrachloride: A halogenated hydrocarbon with anaesthetic properties. It has no medicinal use but is a common industrial solvent. It is particularly toxic to the liver.

Cardiac tamponade: Compression

of the heart by the rapid accumulation of fluid in the pericardial sac. Cardiac tamponade is usually caused by bleeding into the pericardial cavity due to rupture of the heart or one of the coronary arteries, or by a penetrating wound of the heart.

Cardiomyopathy: A primary disease of the heart muscle.

Cartridge: Syn. round. The complete unit of ammunition consisting of projectile, cartridge case, primer and propellant, and in the case of shotgun ammunition, the shell, pellets and wads (*see* wad).

Cartridge case: A metallic or plastic cylinder of firearm ammunition which contains the propellant and into which the primer and projectile are inserted.

Caspar's rule: "At a tolerably similar temperature the degree of putrefaction present in a body after lying in the open air for one week corresponds to that found in a body after lying in water for two weeks or after lying in the earth in the usual manner for eight weeks". (Johann Ludwig Caspar 1786-1864).

Cellular death: See death.

Centre fire ammunition: Ammunition in which the *primer* is contained in a well, located in the centre of the base of the *cartridge case*.

Cerebrospinal fluid: The clear fluid which is secreted by the choroid plexuses of the brain and which circulates through the venticular system of the brain and through the subarachnoid space of the brain and spinal cord.

Cervix: Syn. cervix uteri. The neck of the uterus connecting the uterine cavity with the vagina and consisting of the external os and internal os.

Choke: A constriction in the muzzle end of a shotgun barrel which narrows the area of scatter of shotgun pellets.

Chromatin: Particulate matter in the nuclei of cells stainable with basic dyes. It is the carrier of genetic information.

sex chromatin: A particle of chromatin present only in cell nuclei of female individuals. It represents one of the X chromosomes and has been used to determine the sex of fragmentary human remains.

Clip: Syn. cartridge clip. A removable magazine of a firearm containing unfired cartridges.

Clot: A soft semi-solid coagulum formed in stagnant blood, its structure being largely determined by gravity. It thus differs from a thrombus (*see* thrombus).

chicken fat clot: A bright yellow layer, consisting predominantly of white blood cells, and forming the uppermost part of a clot. The position of the chicken fat clot has been used in attempts to determine the position of the body after death.

currant jelly clot: A dark red layer, consisting predominantly of red blood cells and forming the lower part of a clot.

post mortem clot: A clot formed in the blood vessels, chambers of the heart or sites of hemorrhage after death.

Clotting: See coagulation.

Coagulation: Syn. clotting. The transformation from a liquid state into a solid or semi-solid mass. Usually applied to the formation of fibrin in blood resulting in a *clot* or a thrombus (*see* thrombus).

Cocaine: Syn. "bernice", "candy",

"coke", "C", "corine", "dust", "flake", "gold dust", "snow", "star dust". An alkaloid from the leaves of the Erythroxylon trees native to Peru and Bolivia. Systemically cocaine is a cerebral stimulant, topically a local anaesthetic. Used illicitly it is usually snuffed in the form of a white powder.

"Cokie": Syn. "coke head". A cocaine addict.

"Cold turkey": A sudden drug withdrawal.

Coma: A state of deep unconsciousness from which the person cannot be aroused. Causes of coma include poisonings, brain injuries, stroke, diabetes and uraemia.

Commotio cerebri: *See* concussion.

Conceptus: *See* fetus, *see* embryo.

Concussion: A diffuse injury to an organ caused by a violent impact. Usually applied to the brain (commotio cerebri).

Congenital aneurysms: *See* aneurysm.

"Connect": Syn. "cop", "hit", "make a meet", "score". To purchase drugs illicitly.

Contact flattening: The flattening of muscles which are in contact with a hard surface during rigor mortis.

Contact ring: *See* grey ring.

Contre coup injury: An injury of an organ occuring on the side opposite to that suffering a blow or impact. The term is usually applied to the brain but other organs such as the skull or the lungs may sustain contre coup injuries.

Contusion: An injury without laceration to the superficial tissues of an organ or the body surface caused by a blunt impact.

Coronary arteries: *See* artery.

Coronary thrombosis: Occlusion of one of the coronary arteries (*see* artery) by a thrombus (*see* thrombus). A common cause of heart attacks.

Corpus delecti: The body or essential nature of a crime. Often used incorrectly to designate the corpse in a case of homicide.

Cot death: *See* crib death.

Cranial sutures: The fibrous lines of union between the bones of the vault of the skull. The gradual disappearance of the cranial sutures is one of the anatomical features upon which the estimate of the age of skeletal remains may be based.

Cranium: That part of the skull which encloses the brain.

Crib death: Syn. cot death, sudden infant death syndrome (S.I.D.S.). Sudden death in apparently well infants, usually between the third and twelveth months of life, with negative or minimal autopsy findings.

Cricoid cartilage: The lowermost cartilage of the larynx (*see* larynx).

Crimp: Syn. rolled crimp. In shotgun ammunition the folded over margins of the shell holding the over shot wad (*see* wad) in place.

star crimp: Syn. pie crimp. A pleated crimp eliminating the need for over shot wad (*see* wad).

Crush syndrome: *See* syndrome.

Cut: Syn. incised wound, slash, slice. A wound caused by a sharp object, usually of metal or glass. The wound is longer than deep and tends to gape. Its edges are usually not contused, distinguishing it from a split.

"Cut": To dilute a drug, usually by an admixture of starch or milk sugar.

Cutis anserina: Syn. goose flesh,

goose pimples. A roughening of the skin caused by the contraction of the erector muscles of the hairs. In the living person it is caused by fear or exposure to cold; in the cadaver it is a manifestation of rigor mortis. The presence of cutis anserina in a body recovered from water was at one time regarded as an indication that death had occurred in the water. This view is no longer held.

Cyanides: Common and extremely poisonous industrial chemicals and constituents of insecticides.

Cyanosis: A bluish or greyish discolouration of the skin and mucous membranes due to the presence of insufficiently oxygenated blood.

Cylinder: The circular magazine of a revolver.

Dactylography: The recording of fingerprints as an aid in identification.

Death: The permanent cessation of all vital functions.

molecular death: Syn. cellular death. The permanent loss by the cell of its functional integrity. The earliest manifestation of molecular death appears to be an irreversible change in the selective permeability of the cell membrane.

somatic death: Syn. clinical death. The permanent cessation of respiration and circulation. Absence of response to external stimuli, of spontaneous muscular movements and lack of brain function as determined by the electroencephalograph have recently been added to the criteria on which the definition of somatic death has been based. Somatic death marks the extinction of the biological and legal personality.

Deciduous teeth: Syn. milk teeth. The first dentition of the child consisting of 20 teeth.

Declaration of Sydney (see Sydney)

Decompression sickness: See caisson disease.

Defence wound: See wound.

Delirium: A state of mental disorientation, usually temporary.

Delusion: A false belief, contrary to reality, which cannot be corrected by reasoning.

Dementia: An irreversible mental deterioration, the end result of many intoxications or nervous disorders.

Dermal nitrate test: See paraffin test.

Diacetyl morphine: See heroin.

Diatoms: One-celled microscopic algae possessing a siliceous wall. Their presence in the lungs and bone marrow of bodies recovered from water has been used in the diagnosis of drowning.

Diphenylamine test: See paraffin test.

Diptera: An order of insects consisting of the true flies, mostly possessing a single pair of wings. The order includes the species Calliphora vomitoria which infests recently dead bodies and the larvae of which feed upon the tissues.

Disinterment: See exhumation.

Distal: Adj. Further from the trunk or from the origin.

"Ditch": The front of the elbow, the cubital fossa.

D.O.A.: Abbreviation for "dead on arrival".

Dorsal: See posterior.

Drowning: Death due to the immersion of the nose and the mouth in water or other fluid.

dry drowning: Asphyxia caused by spasm of the larynx caused by the aspiration of small quantities of fluid.

wet drowning: Drowning due to the aspiration of large quantities of fluid.

Dura mater: The outer and strongest of the three membranes surrounding the brain and spinal cord.

Ecchymosis: An extravasation of blood into the skin, mucous or serous membrane. An ecchymosis is larger than a petechial hemorrhage (*see* petechiae).

Edema: The presence of excess fluid in the tissues. Edema may be localized or involve the entire body.

Ejector: A mechanism which expels the empty cartridge from the firearm after it has been withdrawn from the firing chamber by the extractor (*see* extractor).

Electrocution: Death caused by the passage of an electric current through the body. The usual mechanism of death is *ventricular fibrillation* of the heart or paralysis of the respiratory centre of the brain.

Embalming: A method of preserving the cadaver by preventing autolysis and putrefaction. It usually involves the perfusion of the blood vessels with a fixative and the introduction of such a fluid into the body cavities. Modern embalming also involves the application of chemicals to the external body surface for cosmetic purposes.

Embolism: The plugging of a blood vessel by an embolus (*see* embolus). When used without qualification, the embolus consists of a thrombus (*see* thrombus).

air embolism: Occlusion of blood vessels by bubbles of air which may be introduced into the blood stream by positive pressure or by negative pressure in cases of stab wounds of the neck. Air embolism must be distinguished from putrefactive gas.

amniotic fluid embolism: Embolism by the solid constituents of amniotic fluid (*see* amniotic fluid).

bone marrow embolism: Occlusion of blood vessels by fragments of bone marrow. It may follow extensive fractures or orthopedic operations.

bullet embolism: Embolism by a bullet or bullet fragments.

fat embolism: Occlusion of capillary blood vessels by fat droplets. It is most commonly seen in the vessels of the brain, lungs and kidneys and follows fractures or contusions of adipose tissue.

gas embolism: Embolism by an insoluble gas as may be seen in caisson disease.

pulmonary embolism: Occlusion of the main artery of the lung or its branches by an embolus. A common cause of sudden death.

talcum embolism: Embolism due to particles of talcum powder in the circulation. It occurs when medicinal preparations intended for oral use are injected intravenously and leads to the formation of small foci of inflammation in the lungs (*see* Junkie's lung).

Embolus: A mass of undissolved matter brought by the blood stream and plugging a vessel which is too narrow to permit its passage.

Embryo: Syn. conceptus. The developing child in the uterus during the first trimester of pregnancy.

Epiglottis: A leaf shaped structure situated at the root of the tongue and protecting the opening of the *larynx* during swallowing.

Epiglottitis: An inflammation of the *epiglottis,* a cause of rapid death in young children.

Epilepsy: A group of disorders marked by episodic impairment or loss of consciousness and frequently convulsions.

Epiphyseal injury: Dislocation of the epiphysis of a bone often caused by forceful pulling of an extremity. A common type of injury in the battered child syndrome.

Epiphysis: A part of a bone which is separated from the main part during the period of active growth by a layer of cartilage and which unites with the main part during adolescence and early adult life.

Ethyl alcohol: See alcohol.

Evidence: All the means by which an alleged matter of fact is established or disproved.

trace evidence: Evidence based upon the examination of small amounts of biological materials such as blood or upon specimens of soil, textile fibers etc.

Exhibit: An object admitted in court as evidence.

Exhumation: Syn. disinterment. The recovery of a body from the ground. Usually applied to the removal of a body from a grave for the purpose of medical ex-amination or transportation to another burial site.

Exsanguination: Death due to loss of blood from the circulatory system.

Extractor: A device for removing the fired cartridge from the firing chamber (*see* firing chamber).

Fallopian tubes: Syn. oviducts, uterine tubes. A pair of muscular tubes connecting the region of the ovaries (*see* ovary) to the cavity of the uterus (*see* uterus).

Falx cerebri: A fold of *dura mater* separating the cerebral hemispheres and containing in its base the sagittal venous sinus.

Fat embolism: See embolism.

Fetus: Syn. conceptus. The developing child in the uterus during the second and third trimesters of pregnancy.

Firing chamber: The chamber in a firearm in which the cartridge rests in position to be fired.

Firing pin: A device which strikes and thus ignites the primer in a cartridge.

"Fix": An injection of a narcotic, usually intravenously.

"Floater": A decomposing body recovered from water.

Floating chest: Syn. flail chest. A chest having lost stability as the result of multiple rib fractures. The loose rib fragments interfere with the inspiratory expansion of the lungs.

Fontanelles: Soft spots between the skull bones of a fetus or infant. Normally the newborn infant has two fontanelles, an anterior which closes at the age of about 18 months, and a posterior which closes at 6 weeks.

Forensic: Adj. Applied to the law.

forensic medicine: Syn. legal medicine. Those parts of medical knowledge which are applied to legal problems.

Fouling: The deposition of powder and lubricant residues on the skin surrounding the entrance wound of a bullet or on the inside of the barrel.

Fracture: A break in a bone.

bumper fracture: A fracture of one or both legs below the knee caused by the bumper of a motor vehicle. It is usually a compound fracture (*see* compound fracture).

comminuted fracture: A fracture having several fragments due to splintering of the bone.

compound fracture: A fracture communicating with the outside through a wound.

contre coup fracture: A fracture, usually of the bones of the skull, caused by stress transmitted from the point of impact.

depressed fracture: A fracture, usually seen in the vault of the skull, showing depression of fragments towards the brain.

eggshell fracture: A fracture of a flat bone, such as the base of the skull, showing a number of intercommunicating fracture lines, with or without displacement of fragments.

greenstick fracture: A fracture of the long bones of children in which the bone is partly bent and partly broken and in which there is no loss of continuity of the bone.

hairline fractures A fine linear fracture of a bone, hardly visible with the naked eye and without displacement of bone fragments.

radiating fracture: A fracture of a flat bone showing linear fracture lines radiating from a central point of impact.

Frangible: Adj. Brittle, readily fragmented. Applied to bullets used for gallery shooting which fragment on impact.

Gangrene: The death of a limb or portion of an organ in the living body.

Garrotting: Asphyxia caused by the twisting of a ligature around the neck.

Gauge: The unit of measurement for shotgun bore diameters, disregarding any choke (*see* choke). The gauge is equal to the number of solid lead balls of the bore diameter which weigh one pound.

Gestation: The period of intra-uterine development.

Gettler-Yamakami test: hemodilution test (Chapter 6).

Glottis: The voice-producing part of the larynx (*see* larynx) consisting of the vocal cords and the space between.

Gonzales test: *See* paraffin test.

"Goof balls": *See* barbiturates.

Goose flesh: *See* cutis anserina.

Graze: An abrasion of the skin caused by contact with a rough surface. The direction of the graze may be shown by a sharply demarcated beginning and tags of skin at the end.

Grey ring: Syn. contact ring. A grey discolouration of the margins of an entrance wound caused by the metal of the bullet or by bullet lubricant.

Grooves: *See* rifling.

Gun: A firearm.

"Gun": A syringe.

Haigh: John George Haigh (19-09-1949). Executed for the murder of an elderly woman but confessed to the murder of 5 other persons. He claimed to have drunk the blood of his victims. He attempted to destroy the bodies by immersion into vats of acid. The trial was of interest because of the issue of insanity and the technical difficulty of establishing the identity of the victim.

Hallucination: A false perception by ear, smell or sight which has no basis in reality.

Hallucinogenic drug: A drug producing hallucinations such as L.S.D. or mescaline (*see* mescaline).

Hanging: A type of ligature strangulation in which the constricting force is due to gravity.

Haptoglobins: A group of proteins in blood plasma which have been used in paternity studies.

Hashish: Syn. "hash". The resinous juice of the flowering tops and the upper leaves of the female hemp plant Cannabis sativa, sold in the form of cakes or blocks. Usually smoked in a pipe. Due to its high content of cannabinols it is more potent than marihuana.

Heat exhaustion: Syn. heat prostration. A state of collapse following exposure to high temperatures caused by the loss of body fluids and electrolytes.

Hemolysis: Syn. laking of blood. The disintegration of red blood cells and escape of hemoglobin into the surrounding fluid.

Hemoperitoneum: The presence of free blood in the abdominal cavity.

Hemorrhage: The escape of blood from a blood vessel.

Hemothorax: The presence of free blood in the chest cavity.

Heroin: Syn. "H", "Harry", "horse", "joy powder", "scat", "schmeck", "smack", "shit". Diacetyl morphine. A semi-synthetic narcotic made by the acetylation of morphine (*see* morphine). Sold illicitly as a white powder, usually heavily adulterated with milk sugar or quinine. Usually injected subcutaneously or intravenously but may be smoked or snuffed.

"Hooked": Addicted.

"Hot shot": 1. An accidental fatal overdose of a narcotic.
2. A narcotic to which a poison such as strychnine or cyanide has been added to kill a troublesome addict or informer.

Hydrostatic test: Syn. flotation test. A test used in the recognition of live birth and consisting of observing the buoyancy of the lung tissue on water.

Hymen: Syn. maidenhead. A membrane which partially occludes the external opening of the vagina.

Hyoid bone: A U-shaped bone in the neck above the larynx (*see* larynx). From its central body project the greater and lesser cornua. The latter are frequently broken in cases of manual strangulation.

Hyperkalemia: An abnormally high level of potassium in the blood.

Hypnotic: A drug which induces sleep.

Hypostasis: The settling of blood after death into the dependent parts of the body. In the skin it is manifested as lividity. See also Table 1-3.

Hypothermia: A state of abnormally low body temperature.

Hypoxia: Lack of sufficient oxygen.

Iatrogenic: Adj. Caused by the physician. Usually applied to an illness or injury caused by injudicious therapy.

Icard's test: A classical test for the presence of circulation. Subcutaneously injected fluorescein gradually discolours the surrounding tissues if the circulation is still present. Now obsolete.

Idiosyncrasy: An unusual or individual reaction, usually applied to reactions to drugs.

In mortuo: In the dead body.

In vitro: In the glass, in the test tube, under experimental conditions.

In vivo: In the living body.

Infanticide: The killing of an infant by its mother.

Infarct: The death of a portion of an organ in the living body due to the sudden obstruction of its blood supply.

Instar: A stage in the development of an insect larva (*see* larva).

Ischemia: A state of inadequate blood supply to an organ or tissue.

Jacket: A complete or partial shell of hard metal such as copper or nickel surrounding the soft metal core of a bullet.

"Junk": Narcotics.

"Junkie": Syn. "hop head", "hype". A narcotic addict.

"Junkie's lung": Lungs showing microscopic foci of chronic inflammation caused by the intravenous injection of insoluble materials such as starch granules or talcum powder. Seen in drug addicts. Sudden death due to heart failure has been reported.

Laceration: Syn. rupture, tear. A wound caused by crushing or tearing of the tissues and showing a break in the surface.

Lands: The areas on the inner surface of a firearm barrel which are located between rifling grooves (*see* rifling).

Lanugo hairs: Fine hairs which appear at the end of the sixth month of gestation and cover the fetus during the seventh and eighth months. Lanugo hairs have been shed by the time of birth except in the region of the eyebrows, the eyelids and the scalp. The presence of lanugo hairs in the lungs is evidence of *amniotic fluid embolism*.

Larva: Syn. maggot. A stage in the metamorphosis of certain insects between the egg and the pupa. The larva may moult several times, each stage being known as an instar.

Larynx: Syn. voice box. A hollow muscular and cartilagenous structure lined with mucous membrane and situated between the hyoid bone (*see* hyoid) and the trachea. Its components include the *epiglottis, thyroid cartilage* and *cricoid cartilage*. It contains the vocal cords.

Lateral: Adj. away from the mid line, towards the side.

Lesion: An abnormal change in the structure of a tissue.

Leucocyte: A white blood cell.

Lividity: Syn. livor mortis. A dark red or bluish red discolouration of the surface of the dependent portions of the body due to post mortem stasis of blood.

congestion lividity: Lividity caused by the distension of the skin capillaries by blood.

diffusion lividity: Lividity due

to hemoglobin staining of the dependent portion of the skin. Diffusion lividity tends to be "fixed" in contrast to congestion lividity.

Load: 1. In ammunition for rifled weapons, the weight of the propellant.
2. In shotgun ammunition, the weight of the propellant and shot.

L.S.D.: Syn. "acid". Lysergic acid diethylamide. A hallucinogenic drug occurring in morning glory seeds. Now usually produced synthetically.

Magazine: The part of a firearm in which unfired cartridges are stored. A removable magazine is usually called a clip.

Magnum: Adj. extra large or powerful, as applied to ammunition.

Magnus test: A test for the cessation of circulation. A ligature is firmly tied around a finger. If the circulation has ceased no swelling appears distal to the ligature.

"Mainline": To inject a drug intravenously.

Mallory-Weiss syndrome: *See* syndrome.

Malocclusion: A condition in which the teeth of the upper and lower jaws do not meet properly.

Marbling: The appearance of vascular patterns on the skin after death.

M a r i h u a n a: Syn. marijuana, "gage", "grass", "hay", "hemp", "jive", "loco weed", "Mary Jane", "mess", "pot", "rope", "Texas tea", "weed". The flowering tops and upper leaves of the female hemp plant (Cannabis sativa), usually sold as a coarse powder and smoked in the form of hand rolled cigarettes.

Masochism: Pleasure derived from being treated cruelly.

M.D.A.: Methylenedioxyamphetamine. An amphetamine derivative not available on the legitimate market.

Meconium: The feces of the newborn. The absence of meconium in a normal intestine of a newborn points towards live birth.

Medial: Adj. towards the midline.

Mellanby effect: Syn. acute accommodation. For a given concentration of alcohol in the blood, the degree of clinical intoxication is greater when the blood alcohol level is rising than when it is falling.

Meninges: The three membranes surrounding the brain and spinal cord and comprising the dura mater, the arachnoid and the pia mater.

Meningitis: An inflammation of the meninges.

Mescaline: A hallucinogenic drug derived from the peyote cactus.

Methadone: A synthetic narcotic similar in its effects to morphine and used as a substitute drug in the treatment of narcotic addiction.

Methyl alcohol: *See* alcohol.

Milk teeth: *See* deciduous teeth.

Miscarriage: The expulsion of the fetus, usually in the third trimester of pregnancy.

Morphine: A vegetable alkaloid, the principal constituent of opium (*see* opium). Morphine is a powerful narcotic, analgesic and nervous system depressant with addicting properties.

Mors in tabula: Death on the operating table.

Mugging: Syn. yoking. A form of strangulation by means of an arm thrown around the victim's neck from behind.

Mummification: The drying of a

dead body or parts thereof to a brown, leathery, parchment-like condition on exposure to a warm and dry environment.

Muzzle: The forward end of the barrel of a firearm.

Muzzle velocity: The velocity at which a projectile leaves the barrel of a firearm, expressed in feet or meters per second.

Myocarditis: An inflammation of the heart muscle caused by bacteria, viruses, parasites or by hypersensitivity. Myocarditis used to be regarded as a common cause of sudden death; now regarded as rare.

Narcotic: A drug producing stupor, sleep and relief of pain.

Necrosis: The death of cells in the living organism.

Nembutal: A brand of pentobarbital (Abbott Laboratories).

Nembutal capsules, syn. "nimbys", "yellow jackets".

Neurone: A nerve cell.

Obturation: The sealing of powder gases between the cartridge case and the walls of the firing chamber and the bullet and the barrel.

Occiput: The back of the head or skull.

Odontology: Syn. dentistry. The knowledge of the development, structure and function of the teeth as well as of the pathological processes involving them. The forensic applications of odontology are largely concerned with the identification of individuals.

Oligospermia: An abnormally low number of sperm cells in the semen.

Opium: Syn. "hop", "mud", "tar". The juice of the unripe seed capsules of the poppy plant (Papaver somniferum). The milky juice is dried and the crude opium is sold as a dark brown, gummy substance. Its pharmacological activity is due to a number of alkaloids including *morphine* and codeine. Crude opium is usually smoked in pipes.

Ossification: The transformation of cartilage or fibrous tissue into bone.

centres of ossification: Points of bone formation, an early stage in the development of the skeleton. The presence of certain centres of ossification is an indication of the age of a young individual.

Osteology: The knowledge of the development, structure and function of bones.

Ovary: The female sex gland which secretes sex hormones and in which the *ovum* develops.

Overlaying: The accidental smothering of a young child in bed by a sleeping adult. Overlaying used to be regarded as a common event; now regarded as rare.

Overpowder wad: *See* wad.

Overshot wad: *See* wad.

Ovum: The egg or female reproductive cell which, after fertilization, develops into the embryo.

Paraffin test: Syn. dermal nitrate test, diphenylamine test, Gonzales test. A test for the nitrates and nitrites of gunpowder residues on the skin. Paraffin casts of the skin are treated with a solution of diphenylamine and diphenylbenzidine. The test is no longer regarded as sufficiently specific.

Pathology: Syn. pathologic anatomy. That branch of medicine concerned with the alterations in the structure of tissues caused by disease, ageing or violence. The practice of pathology includes the performance of autopsies.

Pedophilia: S e x u a l interest in children.

Peritoneum: A serous membrane which lines the internal surface of the abdominal walls and envelops the abdominal organs.

Peritonitis: An inflammation of the peritoneum.

Permanent cavity: The track left in the tissue by the passage of a projectile. The diameter of the permanent cavity is usually greater than that of the projectile because of the tissue disruption caused by the temporary cavity.

Petechiae: Syn. petechial hemorrhages, pinpoint hemorrhages. Tiny hemorrhages in the skin, mucous membranes and serous surfaces.

Phalanx: Any one of the small bones of the fingers and toes.

Pharynx: The muscular-membranous tube connecting the cavities of the mouth and nose with the *larynx* and esophagus. The portion of the pharynx above the palate is the nasopharynx, that below the palate the hypopharynx.

Pia mater: The innermost of the three membranes which surround the brain and spinal cord.

"Piece": 1. A hand firearm.
2. A container of drugs.

"Pipe": A large vein suitable for the injection of a narcotic.

Placenta: Syn. afterbirth. A round, flat organ at the site of the implantation of the embryo containing both maternal and fetal blood vessels and through which the embryo receives oxygen and nourishment. The finding of placental tissue is absolute proof of pregnancy.

Pneumothorax: Air in the chest cavity. Air may enter the chest cavity through a tear in the lung or through a wound of the chest wall.

Post mortem: Adj. present or occurring after death.

post mortem changes: Physical and chemical processes which commence immediately after death and eventually lead to the complete disintegration of the body.

post mortem interval: The time between death and the examination of the body.

Posterior: Adj. Syn. dorsal. Behind, to the rear of, facing backwards.

Powder stippling: *See* tattoo.

Primer: An explosive substance in firearm ammunition which is ignited by the percussion of the firing pin and which in turn ignites the propellant.

Propellant: The powder in a cartridge which is ignited by the primer and propels the projectile.

Proximal: Adj. nearer to the trunk or the origin.

Psychosis: A group of severe mental disorders in which there is loss of contact with reality and which are usually characterized by hallucinations.

Ptomaines: A group of toxic substances produced by the breakdown of proteins during putrefaction. Formerly believed to be a cause of food poisoning.

Pulmonary embolism: *See* embolism.

Pupa: The resting stage in the metamorphosis of certain insects, between the larva and the adult form.

Putrefaction: The disintegration of the tissues brought about by bacterial action.

putrefactive gases: Gases evolved in the course of putrefaction, largely hydrogen sulphide, ammonia, methane and carbon dioxide.

Rectum: The terminal portion of the large intestine. It opens to the outside through the anus.

Reye's syndrome: See syndrome.

Rh factor: See Rhesus factor.

Rhesus factor: A group of antigens carried on the red blood cells, first found in the rhesus monkey. Individuals possessing the rhesus factor are said to be "Rh positive".

Rifle: A firearm, normally fired from the shoulder, the barrel of which has rifling on its inner surface.

Rifled slug: See slug.

Rifling: A series of spiral grooves on the inner surface of a firearm barrel, designed to impart a spin to the projectile. The number of grooves and their direction (right or left handed) is one criterion on which a classification of firearms is based.

Rigor mortis: Syn. cadaveric stiffening. A stiffening and contraction of the musculature of the body (both voluntary and involuntary) after death. See also Table 1-4.

Rim fire: Ammunition in which the primer is located in a rim surrounding the base of the cartridge case.

Rolled crimp: See crimp.

Round: See cartridge.

Ruxton: "Buck" Ruxton (1899-1936). Physician practicing in Lancaster, England. Native of India. Convicted of the murder of his wife. Her body and that of her maid had been dismembered and concealed in various locations. The medical evidence was of great interest as it involved the determination of the cause of death and the reconstruction of body stature and identification of the victims on the basis of incomplete, decomposing and mutilated remains.

Sadism: A form of perversion in which pleasure or sexual satisfaction is derived from the infliction of cruelty or pain on another person or an animal.

Sagittal: Adj. in an antero-posterior direction.

Salicylates: A group of drugs used as analgesics, fever-reducing agents and for local application. Salicylates are commonly involved in suicidal poisonings in adults and accidental poisonings in children.

Scald: A surface injury caused by moist heat. In the skin the preservation of hairs distinguishes a scald from a burn.

Seat belt injury: Abdominal injuries sustained by flexion over a seat belt during sudden deceleration. Seat belt injuries include compression fractures of the spine and tears of the bowel and mesentery.

Seconal: Brand of secobarbital (Eli Lilly & Co.).

Seconal capsules: Syn. "pinks", "red birds", "red devils", "seggys".

Secretor: An individual secreting blood group substances in the body fluids and secretions such as milk, saliva and seminal fluid. About 80 per cent of the population are secretors.

Sedative: A drug which allays excitement. Sedatives include the barbiturates, bromides and chloral hydrate. In large doses sedatives may act as *hypnotics*.

Segmentation: Syn. box-car sign.

Numerous transverse interruptions of the blood column in the blood vessels of the eye grounds. It has been regarded as one of the earliest signs of death.

Semen: Syn. seminal fluid. A viscous fluid ejected from the penis during orgasm and consisting of spermatoza derived from the testis and of secretions of the prostate gland and seminal vesicles.

Septicemia: Syn. blood poisoning, sepsis. The presence of pathogenic bacteria in the blood.

Sex chromatin: *See* chromatin.

Shapiro plateau: *See* temperature plateau.

Shock: A condition characterized by pallor, low blood pressure, rapid but shallow pulse and clammy perspiration.

primary shock: Syn. faint, syncope. A transient loss of consciousness due to fear or violent emotion.

secondary shock: Syn. oligemic shock, surgical shock, traumatic shock. A state of shock, often progressing to death, caused by a sudden reduction of circulating blood volume.

"Shoot": Syn. "bank", "crank", "drop", "hit", "job". To inject a drug, usually intravenously.

Shot pellets: Pellets of lead or lead alloy in shotgun ammunition.

chilled shot: Especially hardened shot pellets.

Singeing: Syn. branding. An area of burned skin surrounding the entrance wound of a bullet fired at close range and caused by hot gases escaping from the muzzle.

Slug: Syn. rifled slug. A solid projectile made of lead or lead alloy for a smooth bore gun. Slugs have engraved rifling to provide spin and thus ballistic stability.

Smothering: Asphyxia caused by the occlusion of the mouth and nostrils.

Smudging: An area of blackening produced by powder gases and surrounding the entrance wound of a bullet fired at close range.

Somatic death: *See* death.

"Soup": Syn. "hokus". A solution of a narcotic ready for injection.

Spacer wad: *See* wad.

"Speed": *See* amphetamines.

"Speed ball": A combination of a nervous system stimulant (e.g. cocaine) with a depressant (e.g. morphine).

Split: A wound of the skin caused by the compression of the tissue between a hard, blunt object or hard surface and bone. Its edges are contused and there may be "bridging" of the defect, distinguishing it from a cut.

Sprain: The twisting or straining of a joint with injury to the joint capsule or ligaments but without displacement of the bones.

Steering wheel injury: An injury caused by the impact of the steering wheel on the chest and upper abdomen of the driver during sudden deceleration. Common steering wheel injuries include rupture of the liver and a "floating chest".

Stillbirth: The birth of a dead infant during the last trimester of pregnancy or at term. An infant is regarded as stillborn if it has not shown any signs of life while completely external to the mother.

Strangulation: Death caused by compression or constriction of the neck.

ligature strangulation: Strangulation by an object such as a rope, a stocking or a towel.

manual strangulation: S y n .

throttling. Strangulation by one or both hands. Manual strangulation often causes injury to the hyoid bone or thyroid cartilage.

Strychnine: A vegetable alkaloid obtained from the seeds of Strychnos nux vomica. It is a strong nervous system stimulant and convulsant.

Stud gun: A gun firing a bolt, nail or rivet by means of an explosive charge.

Stun gun: A gun firing a captive bolt. Used in the slaughtering of cattle.

Subarachnoid hemorrhage: Hemorrhage between the arachnoid mater and the pia mater. It may be caused by injury or by rupture of a berry aneurysm.

Subdural hemorrhage: Hemorrhage between the dura mater and the arachnoid mater, usually of traumatic origin.

Subluxation: A partial dislocation of a joint.

Superfecundation: The fertilization on two separate occasions of ova produced during the same menstrual cycle.

Superfetation: The fertilization of an ovum in a uterus which already contains a developing embryo.

Sydney, Declaration of: A statement made by the 22nd World Medical Assembly in Sydney, Australia, in 1968. It affirmed that the determination of death should be the responsibility of the physician and should be based upon the usual clinical criteria supplemented by the electroencephalograph. In cases in which the patient was considered as a possible organ donor, the point of death should be ascertained by two physicians who should in no way be concerned with the performance of the subsequent transplantation.

Syncope: *See* shock.

Syndrome: A set of signs and symptoms which occur together.

crush syndrome: Kidney failure caused by severe crushing injuries, usually of the extremities. A similar syndrome may follow the transfusion of incompatible blood.

Mallory - Weiss syndrome: The vomiting of blood due to a tear in the lower esophagus.

Reye's syndrome: A usually fatal syndrome in infants and young children consisting of hyper-excitability, seizures, fatty liver and low blood sugar.

Talcum embolism: *See* embolism.

Tamponade: *See* cardiac tamponade.

Tandem bullet: A military type of ammunition in which two projectiles are placed in sequence in a single round. The tandem bullet is so designed that the two projectiles strike the target separated by a distance.

Tardieu spots: Small pin - point hemorrhages on the pleural surfaces of the lungs, on the heart and other organs which were at one time regarded as diagnostic of asphyxia.

Tattoo: 1. The introduction of insoluble pigments into the skin. Tattoos may be for decorative or identification purposes or accidental.
2. Syn. powder stippling. An area of burned or partially burned powder grains near the entrance wound of a bullet fired at close range.

Temperature plateau: The period immediately after death during which the internal body temperature does not fall. The temperature plateau may last 1 to 5 hours.

Temporary cavity: A momentary cavity created in the tissues by the rapid passage of a projectile. The size of the temporary cavity depends on the energy of the projectile and on its rate of retardation.

Tentorium cerebelli: A fold of *dura mater* separating the cerebrum from the cerebellum.

Thallium: A metal, an ingredient of mouse and rat poisons. It is very toxic. Poisoning is characterized by nervous symptoms and loss of hair.

T. H. C.: Tetrahydrocannabinol, an active constituent of *hashish* and marihuana (*see* marihuana).

Thrombosis: T h e formation or presence of a thrombus (*see* thrombus).

coronary thrombosis: Thombosis narrowing or occluding a coronary artery (*see* artery).

Thrombus: A solid, brittle coagulum formed in circulating blood within blood vessels or chambers of the heart, its structure being largely determined by the turbulence of the blood. Its architecture thus differs from that of a clot (*see* clot).

mural thrombus: A thrombus attached to the wall of a blood vessel or heart chamber.

Thyroid cartilage: The main cartilage of the larynx (*see* larynx). It has two posterior projections on either side, the superior and inferior cornua. The thyroid cartilage is frequently broken during manual strangulation.

Toxic: Adj. pertaining to or acting as a poison.

Toxicology: The science of the nature of poisons, their effects and detection.

Toxin: A poisonous substance produced by bacteria, animals or plants.

Trachea: Syn. windpipe. A cartilaginous tube connecting the *larynx* with the bronchi.

Tracheotomy: Syn. tracheostomy. A surgical operation making an opening into the trachea in the neck to facilitate breathing.

"Track": Syn. "tracer". A linear scar of the skin, often pigmented and situated over veins. See in addicts who inject drugs intravenously.

Trauma: A wound or injury.

traumatic asphyxia: *See* asphyxia.

Tuinal: Brand of secobarbital and amobarbital (Eli Lilly and Co.).

Tuinal capsules: Syn. "double trouble", "rainbows", "tooies".

Twist: The inclination of *rifling* grooves to the axis of the bore of a firearm barrel. Expressed in terms of inches or centimeters of barrel length for one complete turn of the grooves.

Ulcer: An open sore of skin or mucous membrane.

Umbilical cord: A cord connecting the navel of the fetus with the placenta and containing two arteries and one vein.

Uterine tubes: See fallopian tubes.

Uterus: Syn. womb. A hollow muscular organ in the female in which the embryo develops.

Vagal inhibition: Syn. vagus reflex. Stoppage of the heart beat through stimulation of the vagus nerve. Vagal inhibition may be caused by pressure on the neck, immersion in cold water and minor surgical procedures.

Vagina: The tubular musculo-fibrous passage in the female connecting the *vulva* with the cervix (*see* cervix).

Vagus: The tenth cranial nerve originating in the brain stem, passing through the neck and the chest and supplying branches to the larynx, heart, lungs, stomach and abdominal organs.

Vein: A blood vessel carrying blood on its way from the tissues to the heart.

Ventral: *See* anterior.

Ventricles: 1. The two lower chambers of the heart.
2. Four intercommunicating cavities in the brain into which the cerebro-spinal fluid is secreted.

Ventricular fibrillation: Irregular and ineffective contractions of the ventricles of the heart leading to sudden death.

Vernix caseosa: A greasy, greyish-white substance covering the skin of the fetus.

Viability: As applied to a fetus, the stage of development at which it would be capable of an extra-uterine existence. Variously given as 20 to 28 weeks of gestation.

Virtual cooling time: The time the internal body temperature takes to fall through the first 85% of the difference between the body temperature at death and that of the environment. The virtual cooling time has been used in the calculation of the time of death.[50]

Vital: Adj. Characteristic of or essential to life.

vital reaction: A reaction in a tissue such as inflammation, occurring during life and used to distinguish pre mortem from post mortem wounds.

vital signs: Physical signs such as respiration and pulse indicative of the presence of life.

Vulva: The external female sexual organs consisting of the vestibule, clitoris, labia majora and labia minora.

Wad: A disc of felt, cardboard or plastic used in shotgun ammunition.

filler wad: Syn. spacer wad. A felt wad located between the overpowder and undershot wads.

overpowder wad: Syn. base wad. A cardboard wad above the powder load of a shotgun shell.

overshot wad: A thin cardboard wad above the shot held in position by the crimp (*see* crimp). Not present in ammunition having a star crimp (*see* crimp).

plastic one-piece combination wad: In modern shotgun ammunition a single plastic wad located under the shot and taking the place of the filler wad.

Waschhaut: Syn. washerwoman's hands. A wrinkling of the skin of the hands caused by prolonged exposure to moisture. It may occur before or after death.

Whiplash injury: An injury to the tissues of the neck caused by a sudden overextension of the cervical spine. It is common in rear end collisions. The injury usually involves the muscles and spinal ligaments but in severe cases may damage the intervertebral discs, esophagus and trachea.

Widmark's method: A method of determining the alcohol content of biological fluids, based upon the oxidation of the alcohol by acid dichromate and the estimation of excess dichromate.

Womb: *See* uterus.

Wound: A disruption of a tissue caused by violence.

defence wound: A wound on the fingers, hands or forearms of the victim of an attack with a sharp weapon, sustained while trying to grasp or ward off the blade.

hesitation wound: Tentative stabs or cuts made by a suicide prior to the infliction of a lethal wound.

penetrating wound: A wound which extends into an organ or tissue, having an entrance opening only.

perforating wound: A wound which completely transverses an organ or tissue, having both an entrance and exit opening.

Yaw: The angle between the longitudinal axis of a projectile and its line of flight.

BIBLIOGRAPHY

1. Accident Fatalities — Canada 1974. Canada Safety Council, Ottawa, Ontario.
2. Adams EG, Wraxall BG: Phosphates in body fluids. The differentiation of semen and vaginal secretion. For Sci 3:57-63, 1974.
3. Adelson L: A microscopic study of dermal gunshot wounds. Amer J Clin Path 35:393-402, 1961.
4. Algeri EJ: The determination of barbiturate after putrefaction. J For Sci 2:443-455, 1957.
5. Alha AR, Tamminen V: Fatal cases with an elevated urine alcohol but without alcohol in the blood. J For Med 11:3-5, 1964.
6. Backwinkel KD: Injuries from seat belts. J Amer Med Ass 205:305-308, 1968.
7. Baker SP, Spitz WV: Age effects and autopsy evidence of disease in fatally injured drivers. J Amer Med Ass 214:1079-1088, 1970.
8. Balduzzi PC, Greendyke RM: Sudden unexplained death in infancy and viral infections. Pediatrics 38:201-206, 1966.
9. Bardzik S: The efficiency of methods of estimating the time of death by pharmacological means. J For Med 13:141-143, 1966.
10. Beck CS: Contusions of the heart. J Amer Med Ass 104:109-114, 1935.
11. Beck WN: (Changes in the blood alcohol level during combustion and the inhalation of hot gases) (Ger) Deutsch Z Ges Gerichtl Med 33:95-102, 1935.
12. Berg S: (A vital reaction specific for hanging) (Ger) Deutsch Z Ges Gerichtl Med 42: 158-163, 1952.
13. Berg S: (The appearance of tissue hormones in the blood in asphyxia) (Ger) Proc 5th Int Kongr Int Akad f Ger u Soc Med. Vienna, 1961.
14. Berg S: Medico-biological interpretation of sexual delinquency. J for Med 4:82-89, 1957.
15. Berghaus G, Reifenberg U, Dotzauer G: (Determination of sex on skeletal parts) (Ger) J Leg Med 72:255-268, 1973.

16. Beveridge GW, Lawson AAH: Occurrence of bullous lesions in acute barbiturate intoxication. Brit Med J 1:835-837, 1965.
17. Bianchi L, Ohnacker H, Beck K et al.: Liver damage in heat stroke and its regression. Hum Path 3:237-248, 1972.
18. Birkinshaw VJ, Gurd MR, Randall SS: Investigations in a case of murder by insulin poisoning. Brit Med J 2:463-468, 1958.
19. Birrell JH: Safety belts for motor vehicles in Victoria. Med J Austral 1:63-67, 1964.
20. Bogusz MB, Guminska M, Markiewicz J: Studies on the formation of endogenous ethanol in blood putrefying in vitro. J For Med 17:156-168, 1970.
21. Brinkmann B, Jobst U: (Determination of nuclear sex on biological traces) (Ger) J Leg Med 73:1-6, 1973.
22. "Bulletin" Food and Drug Directorate. Dept. of National Health and Welfare. Government of Canada. 2:No. 8, 1971.
23. Caffey J: Multiple fractures in long bones of infants suffering from chronic subdural haematoma. Amer J Roentgenl 56:163-173, 1946.
24. Cameron JM, Johnson HRM, Camps FE: The battered child syndrome. Med Sci Law 6:2-21, 1966.
24. Campbell O'F: Motor cycle accidents in the Ottawa area, 1967. Traffic Injury Research Foundation of Canada, Ottawa.
26. Campbell O'F: Alcohol involvement in fatal motor vehicle accidents 1966-1969. Modern Med of Canada 26:7-10, 1971.
27. Camps FE: Medical and scientific investigations in the Christie case. Medical Publications, London, 1953.
28. Camps FE, Hunt AC: Pressure on the neck, J For Med 6:116-135, 1959.
29. Camps FE: Alcohol. J Roy Coll Phys Lond 2:311-326, 1968.
30. Carpenter HM, Wilkins RM: Autopsy bacteriology. Review of 2,033 cases. Arch Path 77:73-81, 1964.
31. Cimbura G, McGarry E, Daigle J: Toxicological data for fatalities due to carbon monoxide and barbiturates in Ontario. A 4-year survey 1965-1968. J For Sci 17:640-644, 1972.
32. Courville CB, Myers RO: Effects of extraneous poisons on the nervous system — III The asphyxiant gases. Bull Los Angeles Neurol Soc 19:197-223, 1954.
33. Courville CB: The process of demyelination in the central nervous system — IV Demyelination as a delayed residual of carbon monoxide asphyxia. J Nerv Ment Dis 125:534-546, 1957.
34. Cowan ME, Purdon PL: A study of the paraffin test. J For Sci 12:19-36, 1967.
35. Curry AS: Advances in Forensic and Clinical Toxicology. CRC Press, Cleveland, Ohio, 1972.
36. Davidson WM: Sexing from cells. J For Med 7:14-17, 1960.

37. Davies A, Wilson E: The persistence of seminal constituents in the human vagina. For Sci 3:45-55, 1974.

38. Davis JH: Fatal underwater breath holding in trained swimmers. J For Sci 6:301-306, 1961.

39. Dines DE, Baker WG, Scantland WA: Aspiration pneumonitis — Mendelson's syndrome. J Amer Med Ass 176:229-231, 1961.

40. Doering G, Korinth E, Schmidt O: Postmortem glycogenolysis in muscle. J For Med 9:106-115, 1962.

41. Dominguez AM: Problems of carbon monoxide in fires. J For Sci 9:379-392, 1962.

42. Dominguez AM, Halstead JR, Domanski TJ: The effect of postmortem changes on carboxyhaemoglobin. J For Sci 9:330-341, 1964.

43. Dunnett N, Kimber KJ: Urine-blood alcohol ratio. For Sci Soc J 8:15-24, 1968.

44. Durlacher SH, Meier JR, Fisher RS et al.: Sudden death due to pulmonary fat emboli in chronic alcoholics with fatty livers. J For Sci 4:215-228, 1959.

45. Enos WF, Mann GT, Dolan WD: A laboratory procedure for the identification of semen — A preliminary report. Amer J Clin Path 39:316-320, 1963.

46. Evans WED: Adipocere formation in a relatively dry environment. Med Sci Law 3:145-153, 1963.

47. Falconer MA, Taylor DC: Driving after temporal lobectomy for epilepsy. Brit Med J 1:266-269, 1967.

48. Fatteh A: Histochemical distinction between antemortem and post mortem skin wounds. J For Med 11:17-27, 1966.

49. Fazkas IG, Viragas KE: (The content of free histamine in the strangulation mark in hanging as a vital reaction). (Ger) Deutsch Z Ges Gerichtl Med 56:250-268, 1965,

50. Fiddes FS, Patten TD: A percentage method of representing the fall in body temperature after death. Its use in estimating the time of death. J For Med 5:2-15, 1958.

51. Fisher IL: Chloride determination of heart blood. Its use for the identification of death by drowning. J For Med 14:108-112, 1967.

52. Froggatt P, Lynas MA, MacKenzie G: Epidemiology of sudden unexpected death in infants ("cot death") in Northern Ireland. Brit J Prev Soc Med 25:119-134, 1971.

53. Galatius—Jensen F: The use of serum haptoglobin patterns in cases of disputed paternity. Methods of Forensic Science. F. Lundquist, Ed., Vol. 1, Interscience Publishers, New York, 1962.

54. Gee DJ: A case of spontaneous combustion. Med Sci Law 5:37-38, 1965.

55. Geertinger P: Cot deaths associated with congenital anomalies of the parathyroids of infants. J For Med 14:46-59, 1967.

56. Gettler AO, Mattice MR: The "normal" carbon monoxide content of the blood. J Amer Med Ass 100:92-97, 1933.
57. Gibson AG: Alcohol can be absorbed through the respiratory tract. A case report. Med Sci Law 15:64, 1975.
58. Giles E, Elliot O: Race identification from cranial measurements. J For Sci 7:147-157, 1962.
59. Glob PV: The Bog People. Paladin, London, 1971.
60. Gold E, Carver DH, Heineberg H et al.: Viral infection. A possible cause of sudden unexpected death in infants. New Engl J Med 264:53-60, 1961.
61. Gonzales TA, Vance M, Helpern M, Umberger CS: Legal Medicine, Pathology and Toxicology. 2nd ed. Appleton, Century, Crofts, New York, 1954.
62. Gordon EB: Carbon monoxide encephalopathy. Brit Med J. 1:1232, 1965.
63. Gore I, Isaacson HN: The pathology of hyperpyrexia. Observations at autopsy in 17 cases of fever therapy. Amer J Path 25:1029-1046, 1949.
64. Gormsen H: Yeast and the production of alcohol postmortem. J For Med 1:170-171, 1954.
65. Gormsen H: Alcohol production in the dead body. J For Med 1:314-315, 1954.
66. Graham RE: Sudden death in young adults in association with fatty liver. Bull Johns Hopk Hosp 74:16-25, 1944.
67. Grattan E, Jeffcoate G: Medical factors and road accidents. Brit Med J 1:75-79, 1968.
68. Grattan E, Hobbs JA: Injuries to hip joint in car occupants. Brit Med J 1:71-73, 1969.
69. Grob HS: Cytologic sexing. In Personal Identification in Mass Disasters. TD Stewart, Ed. Nat Mus Nat Hist Smithsonian Inst Washington, 1970.
70. Grove SS: Causes of death in the perinatal period. J For Med 6:43-52, 1959.
71. Gustafson G: Forensic Odonotology. American Elsevier Publishing Co. Inc. New York, 1966.
72. Guttman AB, Guttman EB: Acid phosphatase and functional activity of the prostatic (man) and preputial (rat) glands. Proc Soc Exp Biol Med 39:529-532, 1938.
73. Hale HW, Martin JW: Myocardial contusion. Amer J Surg 93:558-564, 1957.
74. Hamilton JB: Seat belt injuries. Brit Med J 4:485-486, 1968.
75. Harris CJJ: Note of carbon monoxide poisoning at the Whitehaven pit disaster. Lancet 4:1693, 1910.
76. Harvey EN, McMillen JH, Butler EG et al.: Mechanism of wounding. In Wound Ballistics. Office of the Surgeon General, Department of the Army, Washington, D.C., 1962.

77. Harvey W, Butler O, Furness J et al.: The Biggar murder. For Sci Soc J 8:155-219, 1968.
78. Harvey WP, Levine SA: Paroxysmal ventricular tachycardia due to emotion. Possible mechanism of death from fright. J Amer Med Ass 150: 479-480, 1952.
79. Hawke et al.: Practical Physiological Chemistry. 12th ed. 1947, cited in Documenta Geigy, 6th ed. 1963.
80. Hebert DC: Safety belts for motor vehicles in Victoria. Med J Austral 1: 67-72, 1964.
81. Hebold G: (Postmortem diffusion of alcohol through the wall of the stomach) (Ger) Deutsch Z Ges Gerichl Med 47:619-624, 1958.
82. Heise HA: Concentrations of alcohol in samples of blood and urine taken at the same time. J For Sci 12:454-462, 1967.
83. Hirsch CS, Adelson L: Absence of carboxyhemoglobin in flash fire victims. J Amer Med Ass 210:2279-2280, 1969.
84. Hirsch CS, Adelson L: Ethanol in sequestered hematomas. Amer J Clin Path 59:429-433, 1973.
85. Hirvonen J, Tiisala R, Uotila U et al.: Roentgenological and autopsy studies on the gas content of the lungs and gastro-intestinal tract in living and stillborn infants and sources of error in resuscitation. Deutsch Z Ges Gerichtl Med 65:73-86, 1969.
86. Huelke DF: Identification of injury mechanisms in automobile crashes. Legal Medicine Annual 1973. Cyril H Wecht, Ed. Appleton, Century, Crofts, New York.
87. James TN: Sudden death in babies. New observations in the heart. Amer J Cardiol 22:479-506, 1968.
88. Jetter WW, McLean R: Poisoning by the synergistic effect of phenobarbital and ethyl alcohol. Arch Path 36:112-122, 1943.
89. Johnstone JM, Lawy HS: Role of infections in cot deaths. Brit Med J 1:706-709, 1966.
90. Jones HD: Medicolegal disinterments. J For Sci 7:363-370, 1962.
91. Kerley ER: Estimation of skeletal age after about age 30. In Personal Identification in Mass Disasters, TD Stewart, Ed. Nat Mus Nat Hist, Smithsonian Inst, Washington D.C., 1970.
92. Kevorkian J: The fundus oculi as a post-mortem clock. J For Sci 6:261-272, 1961.
93. Kind SS: The acid phosphatase test. In Methods of Forensic Science, Vol. 3. AS Curry, Ed. Interscience Publishers, London, New York, 1964.
94. Knight B: Methods of dating skeletal remains. Med Sci Law 9:247-252, 1969.
95. Krishnan SS: Determination of gunshot firing distances and identification of bullet holes by neutron activation analysis. J For Sci 12:112-122, 1967.

96. Krogman WM: A guide to the identification of human skeletal remains. FBI Law Enforc Bull 8:1-29, 1939.
97. Laves W; (Rigor mortis) (Ger) Deutsch Z Ges Gerichtl Med 39:186-198, 1948.
98. Laves W: (The plasma-nucleotide phenomenon in the blood in hypoxia) (Ger) Munch Med Wschr 98:1-4, 1956.
99. Light FW: Gunshot wounds of entrance and exit in experimental animals. J Trauma 3:120-128, 1963.
100. Lister RD, Milson BM: Car seat belts. An analysis of the injuries sustained by car occupants. Practitioner 191:332-340, 1963.
101. Lorenzen GA, Lawson RL: A possible new approach for determining the post mortem interval. J Crim Law Criminol Pol Sci 62:560-563, 1971.
102. Lothe F: The use of larval infestation in determining the time of death. Med Sci Law 4:113-115, 1964.
103. Luke J, Helpern M: Sudden unexpected death from natural causes in young adults. Arch Path 85:10-17, 1968.
104. Luke JL: Strangulation as a method of homicide. Arch Path 83:64-70, 1967.
105. Luvoni R, Marozzi E: Ethyl alcohol distribution in the various organs and fluids of cadavers. J For Med 15: 67-70, 1968.
106. Malamud N, Haymaker W, Custer RP: Heat stroke — a clinicopathologic study of 125 fatal cases. Milit Med 99:397-449, 1946.
107. Mann GT: Sudden death with fatty livers. Med Leg Bull No. 138. Off Chief Med Examin Commonw Virginia.
108. Mant K: Autopsy diagnosis of accidental hypothermia. J For Med 16: 126-129, 1969.
109. Mant K: Sudden death due to acute sickling. Med Sci Law 7:135-136, 1967.
110. Marshall TK, Hoare FE: Estimating the time of death. The rectal cooling after death and its mathematical expression. J For Sci 7:56-81, 1962.
111. Marshall TK: Estimating the time of death. The use of the cooling formula in the study of postmortem cooling. J For Sci 7:189-222, 1962.
112. Marshall TK: The use of the body temperature in estimating the time of death and its limitations. Med Sci Law 9:178-182, 1969.
113. Mason JK, Blackmore DJ: Experimental inhalation of ethanol vapour. Med Sci Law 12:205-208, 1972.
114. May J: (Relation between the concentration of carbon monoxide in the air and the carboxyhaemoglobin content of the blood) (Ger). Arch Gewebepath Gewerbehyg 10:97-105, 1940.
115. Maynert EW, VanDyke HB: The absence of localization of barbital in divisions of the central nervous system. J Pharmac Exp Therap 18:184-187, 1950.

116. McCloskey KL, Muscillo GC, Noordewier B: Prostatic acid phosphatase activity in the postcoital vagina. J For Sci 20:630-636, 1975.

117. McKern TW: Estimation of skeletal age. From puberty to about 30 years of age. In Personal Identification in Mass Disasters. TD Stewart, Ed. Nat Mus Nat Hist Smithsonian Inst Washington D.C. 1970.

118. Mégnin P: (The Fauna of Cadavers — The Application of Entomology in Legal Medicine) (Fre) G. Masson, Paris, 1894.

119. Mendelson CL: Aspiration of stomach contents into lungs during obstetric anaesthesia. Amer J Obstet Gynec 52:191-205, 1946.

120. Mithoefer JC, Mead G, Hughes JMB et al.: A method of distinguishing death due to cardiac arrest from asphyxia. Lancet 2:654-656, 1967.

121. Modell JH: Resuscitation after aspiration of chlorinated fresh water. J Amer Med Ass 185:103-107, 1963.

122. Mole RH: Fibrinolysin and the fluidity of the blood post mortem. J Path Bact 60:413-427, 1948.

123. Montanari GD, Viterbo B, Montanari GR: Sex determination of human hair. Med Sci Law 7:208-210, 1967.

124. Moritz AR, Zamcheck N: Sudden and unexpected deaths of young soldiers. Arch Path 42:459-494, 1946.

125. Moser RH: Diseases of Medical Progress. A Study of Medical Progress. A Study of Iatrogenic Disease. 3rd ed. Charles C. Thomas, Springfield, Illinois, 1969.

126. Mosinger M, Fiorentini H, Depieds R et al.: (The pathology of the asphyxias) (Fre) Ann Méd Lég 41:209-233, 1961.

127. Mueller B: (Death due to drowning) (Ger) Deutsch Z Ges Gerichtl Med 41:400-404, 1952.

128. Neidhart DA, Greendyke RM: The significance of diatom demonstration in the diagnosis of death by drowning. Amer J Clin Path 48:377-382, 1966.

129. Newsletter Vol. 4 No. 2, Traffic Injury Research Foundation of Canada, 1971.

130. Nicholls LC: The Scientific Investigation of Crime. Butterworth & Co. (Publishers) Ltd. London, 1956.

131. Parker DW: The hazards of scuba diving. Canad J Pub Health 56:292-296, 1965.

132. Payne JP, Foster DV, Hill DW et al.' Observations on the interpretation of blood alcohol levels derived from analysis of urine. Brit Med J 3:819-823, 1967.

133. Perkons AK, Jervis RE: Application of radio-activation analysis in forensic investigations. J For Sci 7:449-464, 1962.

134. Peterson B, Petty CS: Sudden natural death among automobile drivers. J For Sci 7:274-285, 1962.

135. Petty CS: Firearms injury research. The role of the practising pathologist. Amer J Clin Path 52:277-288, 1969.
136. Pieczarkowski M: Late post-mortem demonstration of carbon monoxide. Polska Gaz Lek Lwow 16:24, 1937 Abstr. in J Amer Med Ass 108:770, 1937.
137. Pinto FC: For the defence — acid phosphatase. J For Med 6: 147-159, 1959.
138. Pinto FC: Personal communication.
139. Plueckhahn VD, Ballard B: Diffusion of stomach alcohol and heart blood alcohol concentration at autopsy. J For Sci 12: 463-470, 1967.
140. Plueckhahn VD, The significance of blood alcohol levels at autopsy. Med J Austral 4:118-124, 1967.
141. Pollak OJ: Semen and seminal stains — a review of methods used in medicolegal investigations. Arch Path 35:140-196, 1943.
142. Ponsold A: Lehrbuch der Gerichtlichen Medizin. Georg Thieme, Stuttgart, 1967.
143. Prinsloo I, Gordon I: Postmortem dissection artefacts of the neck — their differentiation from ante-mortem bruises. South Afric Med J 25:358-361, 1951.
144. Prokop O: (Acid phosphatase in the secretion of helix pomatia) (Ger) Forum Kriminalistik 3:33-34, 1966.
145. Raekallio J: Estimation of the age of injuries by histochemical and biochemical methods. J Leg Med 73:83-102, 1973.
146. Ramsey H, Haag HB: The synergism between the barbiturates and ethyl alcohol. J Pharmac Exp Ther 88: 313-322, 1946.
147. Raventos J: The distribution in the body and metabolic fate of barbiturates. J Pharm Pharmac 6:217-235, 1954.
148. Rees B, Rothwell TJ: The identification of phospho-gluto-mutase isoenzymes in semen stains and its use in forensic case-work investigations. Med Sci Law 15:284-293, 1975.
149. Ringrose CA: Medical assessment of the sexually assaulted female. Med Trial Techn Quart 245-247, 1969 Annual.
150. Rodier J: (Formation of alcohol in the viscera during putrefaction) (Fre) Ann Méd Lég 39:455-461, 1959.
151. Rupp JN: Sperm survival and prostatic acid phosphatase activity in victims of sexual assault. J For Sci 14: 177-183, 1969.
152. Ryan GA: Injuries in traffic accidents. New Engl J Med 276: 1066-1076, 1967.
153. Schwarzacher W: (The mechanism of death due to hanging) (Ger) Deutsch Z Ges Gerichtl Med 11:145-152, 1928.
154. Schwarzfischer F: (Chemical processes during the resolution of rigor mortis) (Ger) Deutsch Z Ges Gericht Med 39:421-428, 1948.
155. Scott W, Root I, Sanborn B: The use of vitreous humor for

determination of ethyl alcohol in previously embalmed bodies. J For Sci 18:913-916, 1974.

156. Seymour FI: Viability of spermatozoa in the cervical canal — preliminary report. J Amer Med Ass 106:1728, 1936.

157. Shapiro HA, Gluckman J, Gordon I: The significance of fingernail abrasions of the skin. J For Med 9:17-19, 1962.

158. Shapiro HA: The post-mortem temperature plateau. J For Med 12:137-141, 1965.

159. Sharpe N: The significance of spermatozoa in victims of sexual offences. Can Med Ass J 89:513-514, 1963.

160. Sigler LH: Emotional disturbance as a cause of an acute cardiac insult. Amer J Cardiol 4:557-562, 1959.

161. Simpson K: Modern Trends in Forensic Medicine. Butterworth & Co. Ltd. London, 1953.

162. Smith FR: Air embolism as a cause of death in scuba diving in the Pacific Northwest. Dis Chest 52:15-20, 1967.

163. Smith HW: Methods of Forensic Science Vol. IV. Interscience Publishers, 1966.

163a. Smith HW: Drinking and driving. Crim Law Quart 3:65-124, 1960-1961.

164. Soutter C: (The level of chlorides in drowning) (Fre) Ann Méd Lég 16:217-243, 1936.

165. Spitz WV: (The diagnosis of drowning by the demonstration of diatoms in organs) (Ger) Deutsch Z Ges Gerichtl Med 56:42-45, 1965.

166. Spitz WV: Essential postmortem findings in the traffic accident victim. Arch Path 90:451-457, 1970.

167. Stoll: (Investigation of the postmortem penetration of carbon monoxide into the body) (Ger) Vierteljschr Gerichtl Med 3F 38:46-50, 1909.

168. Strub CG, Frederick LG: The Principles and Practice of Embalming. Lawrence G Frederick, Publisher, Dallas, 1959.

169. Sturner WQ, Putnam RS: Suicidal insulin poisoning with nine day survival. J For Sci 17:514-521, 1972.

170. Sube J, Ziperman HH, McIver WJ: Seat belt trauma to the abdomen. Amer J Surg 113: 346-350, 1967.

171. Sudden and Unexpected Deaths in Infancy (Cot Deaths). Report of the Proceedings of the Sir Samuel Bedson Symposium, Cambridge, 1970. FE Camps, Ed. Bristol: John Wright & Sons Ltd. 1972.

172. Sunshine I, Hackett E: Chemical findings in cases of fatal barbiturate intoxication. J For Sci 2:149-158, 1957.

173. Sutton RNP, Emery JR: Sudden death in infancy. A microbiological and epidemiological study. Arch Dis Childhood 41:674-677, 1966.

174. Tarsitano F: (Value of the Gettler-Yamakami test for the diagnosis of drowning) (Ital) Arch di Antropol Crim Psich e Med Leg. Milano. 29:17-30, 1949.
175. Taylor's Principles and Practice of Medical Jurisprudence. 8th ed. J & A Churchill, London, 1928.
175a. Taylor's Principles and Practice of Medical Jurisprudence. 12th ed. Keith Simpson, Ed. J & A Churchill, London, 1966.
176. Thermal E: (Histological differentiation of skin blisters due to heat and to poisoning by barbiturates) (Ger) Deutsch Z Ges Gerichtl Med 51:180-189, 1961.
177. Thieme FP: Sex in negro skeletons. J For Med 4:72-81, 1957.
178. Thomas F, VanHecke W, Timperman J: The detection of diatoms in the bone marrow as evidence of death by drowning. J For Med 8:142-144, 1961.
179. Thomas DM, Conner EH: Management of the patient overcome by smoke. J Kentucky Med Ass 66: 1051-1056, 1968.
180. Thurston G: Preternatural combustibility of the human body. Med Leg J 29:100-103, 1961.
181. Trotter M, Gleser GC: Estimation of stature from long bones of American whites and negroes. Amer J Phys Anthropol N.S. 10:463-514, 1952.
182. Trube-Becker E: (The assessment of death by hypothermia) (Ger) Deutsch Z Ges Gerichtl Med 59: 211-227, 1967.
183. Tsuchihashi Y: Studies on personal identification by means of lip prints. For Sci 3:233-248, 1974.
184. Walcher K: (Concerning asphyxia) (Ger) Erg Allg Path path Anat 36:63-65, 1943.
185. Walls HJ: Fatal barbiturate poisoning. J For Med 5:27-53, 1958.
186. Weining E, Zink P, Reinhardt G: (Permeability of the human bladder for ethanol) (Ger) J Leg Med 67:147-157, 1970.
187. Wilks SS, Clark RT: Carbon monoxide determinations in post mortem tissues as an aid in determining physiologic status prior to death. J Appl Physiol 14:313-320, 1959.
188. Wilson RA, Savage CM: Restraint system effectiveness. A study of fatal accidents. Automotive Safety Engineer Seminar 1973. Environmental Activities Staff, G. M. Corp. Michigan, U.S.A. cited in "The Human Collision", Ministry of Transportation and Communications, Province of Ontario, 1975.
189. Wooley PV, Evans WA jr.: Significance of skeletal lesions in infants resembling those of traumatic origin. J Am Med Ass 158:539-543, 1955.
190. Young M, Turnbull HM: An analysis of the data collected by the Status Lymphaticus Investigation Committee. J Path Bact 34:213-258. 1931.

INDEX